Beauty Minus The Expense Of A DeadlyPrice

KAREN VINCENT

DEDICATION

I would like to dedicate this book to women all over the world.

CONTENTS

ACKNOWLEDGMENTS

I would like to acknowledge Dr. Melanie Lutner for teaching me several beauty secrets. It is through learning some of her natural beauty secrets, doing extensive research on many other natural beauty alternatives and trying most of them out on myself, I was able to get the experience to share them with the world. I feel very strongly about the beauty secrets that I mention in this book and as a result, I was inspired to write this book. I would also like to acknowledge international beauty guru and beauty expert Anya Zoto for teaching me a whole lot on natural beauty regimes. Anya Zoto is also a cosmetologist, beauty and holistic therapist, hairdresser, lecturer, coach and educator. Last but not least I would like to acknowledge Laura Gordon who is a model and beauty expert. She has taught me beauty secrets that celebrities use and which are very inexpensive and bring quick or almost instant results.

DISCLAIMER

The author of this book is not a beauty expert or a medical doctor. She has no formal medical or beauty training. As a person who loves beauty and has experimented, researched and tried several beauty alternatives for years, she shares in this book some of the beauty secrets she's learned. Before beginning any weight loss programs or trying any or trying anything concerning your health, you should consult with a licensed health care provider and be monitored throughout the entire process. This book is not intended to provide medical advice, diagnose illness, or in any way attempt to practice medicine. It is not intended to replace, personal medical care from a licensed health care practitioner. Doing anything recommended or suggested in this book must be done at your own risk. This book is based on an inspired true story. Most of the things mentioned in this book are things that were taught to the author by actually beauty experts and specialist. In this book she shares most of the things that she has learned about beauty. This book is derived from the author's memory and best recollection of what she's learned during a period of several years of research. Names, dates, locations and actual events may be changed, embellished, exaggerated, or fictionalized for dramatic effect. The author is forced to include this disclaimer due to the litigious nature of today's world, and the expected attacks, criticism, and attempts to suppress and discredit this work.

INTRODUCTION

First I would like to thank you for purchasing my book. Please read this book cover to cover. I have put a lot of time, effort and research into getting you this information. I wrote this book to help women all over the world to achieve beauty without paying the later high price of cancer and other illness associated with using and enduring unnatural or harmful products and procedures. Also I attempt to give women an alternative to be able to use products that they might already have at home in their kitchen or for them to be able to use a beauty alternative that would be very inexpensive and still be able to achieve the same results as they would with expensive and harmful products. In this book I will speak about beauty, Its many effect on society and I will share with you several beauty secrets which I have learned, some of which I have even tried as well. I am a firm believer that beauty shouldn't take much work and we certainly shouldn't have to deal with illnesses derived from trying to achieve this goal. It should come effortlessly, be done in a healthy way and not leave you in debt. In this book I will be focusing on mainly women's beauty issues and how to solve most of these issues in an easy way. I will mention beauty regimes on skin, nails, hair etc. Most importantly I will speak on where the beauty begins which is in our mind. My intentions are to enhance beauty all over the world. I believe that this book not only outline the problem, but it certainly gives you a workable solution to your beauty issues. My goal is to help women all over the world by sharing with them my beauty secrets and beauty regimes that I have researched as well. I'd like to begin a love revolution for women to begin loving themselves unconditionally and embracing their beauty. Also I'd like for women to learn that they can achieve their beauty goals, whatever they may be, without using products that contain harmful ingredients.

1 BEAUTY

"Imperfection is beauty; madness is genius; and it's better to be absolutely ridiculous than to be absolutely boring"

- Marilyn Monroe

You are about to learn about beauty and several regimes to enhance your natural beauty. Also the effect that beauty has on human beings mind and body. So let's get into it You may be surprised to learn your skin is actually your body's largest organ. Not only is it the largest organ accounting for approximately 16% of body weight, but it is also our protective armor. Good health often is reflected in an attractive, youthful appearance and so it is vitally important we look after this 'organ.' Skin is truly amazing, one of the most complex organs in the body.

What is beauty?

Beauty is a characteristic of a person, animal, idea, object, or place that provides a perceptual experience of pleasure or satisfaction. Beauty is studied as part of aesthetics, social psychology, sociology and culture. An "ideal beauty" is an entity which is admired, or possesses features widely attributed to beauty in a particular culture, for perfection. The experience of "beauty" often involves an interpretation of some entity as being in balance and harmony with nature, which may lead to feelings of attraction and emotional well-being. Because this can be a subjective experience, it is often said that "beauty is in the eye of the beholder." There is evidence that perceptions of beauty are evolutionarily determined, that things, aspects of people and landscapes considered beautiful are typically found in situations likely to give enhanced survival of the perceiving human's genes. There is evidence that a preference for beautiful faces emerges early in child development, and that the standards of attractiveness are similar across different genders and cultures. A study published in 2008 suggests that symmetry is also important because it suggests the absence of genetic or acquired defects. Although style and fashion vary widely, cross-cultural research has found a variety of commonalities in people's perception of beauty. The earliest Western theory of beauty can be found in the works of early Greek philosophers from the pre- Socratic period, such as Pythagoras. The Pythagorean school saw a strong connection between mathematics and beauty. In particular, they noted that objects proportioned according to the golden ratio seemed more attractive. Ancient Greek architecture is based on this view of symmetry and proportion. Plato considered beauty to be the idea above all ideas.

Aristotle saw a relationship between beautiful and virtue, arguing that "Virtue aims at the beautiful." During the Gothic era, the classical aesthetical canon of beauty was rejected as sinful. Later, the Renaissance and Humanism rejected this view, and considered beauty as a product of rational order and harmony of proportions. Renaissance artists and architect (such as Giorgio Vasari in his "lives of artists") criticized the Gothic period as irrational and barbarian. This point of view over Gothic lasted until Romanticism, in the 19th century. The 20th century saw an increasing rejection of beauty by artists and philosophers alike, culminating in postmodernism's anti-aesthetics. This is despite beauty being a central concern of one of postmodernism's main influences, Friedrich Nietzsche, who argued that the Will to Power was the Will to Beauty. In the aftermath of postmodernism's rejection of beauty, thinkers have returned to beauty as an important value. American analytic philosopher Guy Circello proposed his New Theory of Beauty as an effort to reaffirm the status of beauty as an important philosophical concept. Elaine Scarry also argues that beauty is related to justice.

Beauty In Humans

The characterization of a person as "beautiful", whether on an individual basis or by community consensus, is often based on some combination of inner beauty, which includes psychological factors such as intelligence, personality, politeness, grace, integrity, charisma, elegance and congruence, and outer beauty (i.e. physical attractiveness) which includes physical attributes which are valued on an aesthetic basis. Standards of beauty have changed over time, based on changing cultural values. Historically, paintings show a wide range of different standards for beauty. However, humans who are relatively young, with smooth skin, well-proportioned bodies, and regular features, have traditionally been considered the most beautiful throughout history. Researchers have replicated the result under more controlled conditions and found that the computer generated, mathematical average of a series of faces is rated more favorably than individual faces. Evolutionarily, it makes logical sense that sexual creatures should be attracted to mates who possess predominantly common or average features. A feature of beautiful women that has been explored by researchers is a waist-hip ratio of approximately 0.70.

Physiologists have shown that women with hourglass figures are more fertile than other women due to higher levels of certain female hormones, a fact that may subconsciously condition males choosing mates. Sad but true and often is a huge mistake. People are influenced by the images they see in the media to determine what is or is not beautiful. Some feminists and doctors have suggested that the very thin models featured in magazines promote eating disorders, and others have argued that the predominance of white women featured in movies and advertising leads to a euro-centric concept of beauty, feelings of inferiority in women of color, and internalized racism. The "black is beautiful" cultural movement has sought to dispel this notion. The concept of beauty in men is known as 'bishonen' in Japan. Bishōnen refers to males with distinctly feminine features, physical characteristics establishing the standard of beauty in Japan and typically exhibited in their pop culture idols. A multi-billion-dollar industry of Japanese aesthetic salons exists for this reason.

The Effects Beauty And Media Has on Society

Beauty presents a standard of comparison, and it can cause resentment and dissatisfaction when not achieved. People who do not fit the "beauty ideal" may be ostracized within their communities. The television sitcom called, "Ugly Betty" portrays the life of a girl faced with hardships due to society's unwelcoming attitudes toward those they deem unattractive. However, a person may also be targeted for harassment because of their beauty. In Malena, a strikingly beautiful Italian woman is forced into poverty by the women of the community who refuse to give her work for fear that she may "woo" their husbands. The documentary "Beauty is in the eye of the beheld explores both the societal blessings and curses of female beauty through interviews of women considered beautiful. Researchers have found that good looking students get higher grades from their teachers than students with an ordinary appearance. Some studies using mock criminal trials have shown that physically attractive "defendants" are less likely to be convicted—and if convicted are likely to receive lighter sentences—than less attractive ones (although the opposite effect was observed when the alleged crime was swindling, perhaps because jurors perceived the defendant's attractiveness as facilitating the crime).

Studies among teens and young adults, such as those of psychiatrist and self-help author, Eva Rivo, show that skin conditions have a profound effect on social behavior and opportunity. How much money a person earns may also be influenced by physical beauty. One study found that people low in physical attractiveness earn 5 to 10 percent less than ordinary looking people, who in turn earn 3 to 8 percent less than those who are considered good looking. Discrimination against others based on their appearance is known as 'lookism.' St. Augustine said of beauty "Beauty is indeed a good gift of God; but that the good may not think it a great good, God dispenses it even to the wicked."

My Own Opinion On Beauty

I think that beauty begins within and if you truly possess beauty within, it will shine through you to enhance your outer beauty to make you a gorgeous human being. However I do believe that if there is something that you would like to change about yourself, you should do it only if it makes you happy. If you decide to enhance your beauty, it should be solely your decision and you should be doing it only for yourself and not for someone else or because you feel that someone will accept you or treat you better as a result of your enhancement. Think about this...

Imagine if everyone in this world were to look the same and possess the same beauty with no unique features or personalities. What a boring world we would live in and dating would be the worst thing ever. I like the fact that we have so many different types of beautiful people on this earth. Our diversities are what makes this world such a wonderful place. It feels good to know that there are so many different cultures to learn from and interact with. The diversity in itself makes for a beautiful world. So in my opinion beauty start from within. Self- love and personality are the foundation for inner beauty and self -love. I also think that if a person wants to enhance their imperfections, they should first love themselves. It's like a person who loves themself but likes to look at their face as a canvas that they apply make up to.

2 SELF - LOVE

Self-love is caring about oneself, taking responsibility for oneself, respecting oneself, and knowing oneself. Loving oneself is being realistic and honest about one's strengths and weaknesses. Being arrogant, conceited and egocentric are often confused with loving oneself. Those are not actually acts of self- love. In order to have the ability to truly love another person, you must first love yourself unconditionally. I think that we have all struggled with this before. Honestly I didn't always love myself and as a result I would meet people who were hateful and mean to me. However after having lived several unfavorable experiences in my life I had to take time off from meaningless "relationships" (sexual and emotional) and find myself. It was a life changing moment for me because it was the beginning of a great discovery within me. I fell in love with myself and thought about how I've sold myself short in the past because I didn't know who I was. So with some soul searching and spending the past few years being single I was able to find love within me for myself. I also found that I have so many different talents and gifts that I never knew I had. So now I love myself unconditionally and know that I know my worth, I will only accept people who appreciate and value my worth. Loving yourself is the first best feeling that you will ever have in your life. Once you love yourself, you should never have an issue with people's opinion about you or your beauty because you know who you are. You will only allow people to treat you the way you believe that you should be treated and you will demand respect. You will embodies confidence and that is not only beautiful but it is also very sexy. There might be people who will say, "oh, she's conceited or he's conceited." Know that they feel that way because they have no idea what it is like to love themselves. If they do not know what self- love feels like, how can they know that what you're feeling for yourself is self- love?

There is a huge difference between being conceited and loving oneself. We are living in a world where the most beautiful people (inside and out) do not have self-love. This worries me because I have a little girl and I couldn't imagine seeing her go through self loathe and all the mental issues that come with that stuff. I am speaking from experience. Beginning to love yourself for the first time is quite a process. If you are just starting this journey of self-love, I advise that you not be in a relationship at this time. If you are in a relationship and you ask you lover for a break and if they love you enough they will understand and give you as much time as you need. You must first find out who you are. Once you know who you are then it makes it a lot easier to love yourself because then you will know why it is that you love yourself and what qualities and features you love about yourself. As time goes by that love becomes stronger and stronger. Then you will become a person of substance and that will make you a truly beautiful person. Automatically once you love yourself, that energy will attract other people who will also love you unconditionally but be careful because it can also attract people who think that they love themselves and that feed off your loving energy. You will know when this happens.

Here Are Examples of Someone With Self and Someone Without Self-Love:

The person with self - love: If I give you a gift, I give it because it's what I want to do and I do it without expectation. If you don't like it I might feel sad or disappointed, but I can accept that's your choice. Either way, I still know that what I did was a kind thing and I still have a good sense of self-love and self-acceptance.

Versus

The person without self- love: If I give you a gift, I give it because it's what I want to do, but I do it wanting you to like it and, by association, like me (with expectation). If you like it and praise me, I might feel warm and good about myself. If you don't like it I might feel very sad and disappointed, leading to thoughts that I have failed and let you down. My sense of self has decreased because I didn't fulfill my goal of you - liking my gift and giving me love and acceptance back.

Learning to Love Yourself

So why is self-love important and how do I get it?
It helps to realize that you are as important as anyone else, and what you think and feel is valid. For many, this is the most difficult part. Maybe you've grown up thinking that others are always better than you, and you don't matter, and people aren't interested in you unless you please them. But that thinking will only lead you to conclude that others' happiness is more important than yours, and it isn't.

Steps to Self-love

Self-care means you treat yourself just as kindly and thoughtfully as you would anyone else. If you are uncomfortable doing something, then you don't do it and that's OK. Just because somebody might be disappointed that you didn't help him or her, that's his or her choice to feel that way.

Considering your needs

If that means others don't get all of you, all the time, then that's also OK. People can learn to adjust and be responsible for themselves.

Caring for yourself with the same level of effort that you do for others

That might mean you don't always fulfill your goal of helping others because you'd prefer to spend time doing something for yourself. That's not selfish.

Accepting yourself for all that you are, both your positive aspects and your human fallibility

You cannot be all good all the time. That's OK. You can work on self-improvement, but that doesn't mean you discount the parts of yourself you don't like as much. Those aspects are still part of your whole.

Saying no to others' request

That's OK. You are not totally responsible for everybody else's needs. Working toward self-love and acceptance can take time. If you are somebody who has little regard for yourself, then you might want to start with self-like-a-little, working up to self-like. In time, you'll learn to self-love and accept yourself for all that you are.

Cultural Influences

We're taught by society that our worth is found in the idols of our culture, technology, money, attractiveness, and romantic relationships. If you base your self -worth on the external world, you'll never be capable of self-love. Your inner critic will flood you with thoughts of, "I'm not good enough, I don't have enough, and I don't do enough. "Feelings of lack are never-ending. Every time a goal is reached or you possess the next big thing, your ego will move the line. Start to shift Your Self-Perception. Feeling worthy requires you to see yourself with fresh eyes of self-awareness, , and love. Acceptance and love must come from within. You don't have to be different to be worthy. Your worth is in your true nature, a core of love and inner goodness. You are a beautiful light. You are love. We can bury our magnificence, but it's impossible to destroy. Loving ourselves isn't a one - time event. It's an endless, moment by moment ongoing process. It begins with you, enfolding yourself in your own affection and appreciation. Steps to discover your worth and enfold yourself in affection and appreciation. Begin your day with love for yourself. Remind yourself of your worthiness before getting out of bed. Also in the morning you can say to yourself in front of the mirror, "I Love You". Breathe in love and breathe out love. Enfold yourself in light. Saturate your being in love. Take time to mediate and create a daily journal. Spend time focusing inward daily. Begin with 5 minutes of meditation and 5 minutes of journaling each morning. Gradually increase this time. Talk yourself into happiness, it works.

Use affirmations to train your mind to become more positive. Put a wrist band on your right wrist. When you're participating in self-abuse of any form, move the band to your left wrist.

Become emotionally honest with yourself. Let of go of numbing your feelings. Shopping, eating, and drinking are examples of avoid discomfort, sadness, and pain. Mindfully breathe your way through your feelings and emotions. Expand your interests Try something new. Learn a language. Go places you've never been. Do things you haven't done before. You have a right to an awesome life. Enjoy life enhancing activities that make you happy. Find exercise you like to do. Discover healthy foods that are good for you. Turn off technology for a day and spend time doing things that make you feel alive. Become willing to surrender to yourself. Breathe, relax, and let go of all things that do not serve you or make you happy. You can never see the whole picture. You don't know what anything is for. Stop fighting against yourself by thinking and desiring people and events in your life should be different. Your plan may be different from your soul's intentions. Work on personal and spiritual development within yourself. Be willing to surrender and grow. Life is a journey. We are here to learn and love on a deeper level. Take penguin steps and life becomes difficult. One step at a time is enough to proceed forward. Own your potentials and know them. Love yourself enough to believe in the limitless opportunities available to you. Take action and create a beautiful life for yourself. Be patient with yourself , it will come easier as time goes by. Let go of urgency and fear. Relax and transform striving into thriving. Trust in yourself, do good work, and the Universe will reward you. Live in appreciation as much as you can. Train your mind to be grateful. Appreciate your talents, beauty, and brilliance. Love your imperfectly perfect self. Be guided by your intuition. All answers come from within. Look for signs and pay attention to your gut feelings. You'll hear two inner voices when you need to make a decision. The quiet voice is your higher self; the loud voice is your ego. Always go with the quieter voice. Do what honors and respects you.

Don't participate in activities that bring you down. Don't allow toxic people in your life. Love everyone, but be discerning on who you allow into your life. Learn to accept uncertainty. Suffering comes from living in the pain of the past or the fear of the future. Put your attention on the present moment and be at peace. Learn to forgive yourself. Learn from your mistakes and go forward.

Use this affirmation, "I forgive myself for judging myself for _____ (fill in the blank i.e. for getting sick, for acting out, for not doing your best.)

Discover the power of fun. Self-love requires time to relax, play, and create face-to-face interaction with others. Our fast-paced world creates a goal setting, competitive craziness that doesn't leave room for play. Dr. Steve Brow says, "The opposite of play isn't work, it is depression." Be real with others. Speak up and speak out. Allow yourself to be seen, known, and heard. Get comfortable with intimacy. Focus on the positive things. Go to your heart and dwell on and praise yourself for what you get right in all areas. It is very important to become aware of self -neglect and rejection. Become conscious of your choices. Ask yourself several times throughout the day, "Does this choice honor me?" Imagine what your life would look like if you believed in your worth Dedicate your life to loving you. Make it your main event. If you feel the need to seek professional help, it's ok. We all need professional help at times. Self-rejection and neglect is painful. You deserve to be happy. You have a right to be accepted and loved. If necessary, seek help from a support group, counselor, or coach. It's the best investment you can make. We are all interconnected, when I love me, I also love you. Together through our love, we can heal ourselves, each other, and the world. Love is our purpose, our true calling. It begins with and within each of us. By following these steps you should be again to achieve self-love and then you can begin to focus on your inner beauty.

3 INNER BEAUTY

What is inner beauty?

Inner beauty is the most important feature in our human being. All of our actions in a day draw from that inner beauty or soul, if you wish. Have you ever wondered what makes you act the way you do or who you are, inside? Are we are just a collection of cells that happened to come together by chance or is there some grand design someone we can't see or touch that brought us all together? Inner beauty shows itself in many ways perhaps by helping an elderly neighbor with their yard work or volunteering your time to your community. Love is an expression of inner beauty. Does one give love on a daily basis? Does one feel Loved on a daily basis? Hope is a belief in a positive outcome related to events and circumstances in one's life and the lives of others. This can only come from a place of inner beauty. Do you feel compassion toward another human being when you see them in pain or suffering? Compassion comes from inner beauty, at times you can feel it tug at your heart, sometimes you can ignore it but deep down it's always there.

What about outer beauty?

 Can outer beauty, say a beautiful waterfall, a majestic mountain or the brilliant stars in heaven, be enjoyed without inner beauty? I think not. A person can be attracted by outward beauty only to find on closer examination that it is ugly on the inside. A beautiful looking person can be filled with hatred or with love. But how do we know unless we look on the inside? We often judge people when we first meet them by the way they look. It has always been said; you cannot judge a book by its cover. So look inside when you first meet people and look for that inner beauty, in the long run it is far more important than outward beauty. What can physical things in life do for the soul? The answer is "nothing". You need to fill the soul otherwise it starves. Is your inner soul starving?

You can satisfy the hunger with acts of kindness and love, there is plenty in this world to fill the soul. Use it every day and I believe you will be full in no time. After 9/11 I felt love and compassion for all of my fellow Americans, I remember sitting at a toll booth waiting for the person in front of me, fumbling to find the correct change. Any other time I would have been a bit angry at the wait but this time I would have waited all day without anger. I believe it was because we were all one during that time, one country, one people. Why can't it be like that every day as we work, play and live? I don't have all the answers nor do I proclaim to be fault free but I do know the feelings of my own heart. I am sure that each one of us has thought some of these very things at some point in our lives.

I don't want to be on my death bed saying, "I did it all wrong"; there are no do overs. Your inner beauty can flourish and grow, no one can quell it and no one can take it away. When growing up, the quest to be beautiful and maintain beauty is always a constant struggle. Somehow in this generation were there has been a high importance placed on "beauty." Being perceived as beautiful has become a priority. As teenagers we are constantly bombarded with imagery from TV, movies and music that tell the individual that if they do not dress, act, or even have a certain body type they have no hopes to be distinguished as beautiful. This constant exposure is the catalyst for the stress placed on both girls and boys. To them the statement "outward beauty is transient, but inner beauty is lasting" is seen as a cliché that is constantly used by their elders to instill them with confidence in themselves. Seldom do they realize that this so called "overused expression" is of monumental importance and should be considered one of the many laws of life. How many times have we looked in the mirror at our own faces and felt that we didn't measure up to the current standards of beauty?

When we finally turn away from our reflection we end up feeling disheartened. But why is this? The problem is many people let their outward beauty define them, and very few naturally let their inner beauty radiate. While it is true that outer beauty is the very first impression that someone gets when meeting you. It is the inner beauty that we all possess that makes the second and the lasting impression. It is this holistic beauty that is so real, honest and pure that reveals the intricate and complex contents of our souls that cannot be viewed, judged or predetermined by our "outward" complexion.

"Do not let your adorning be external, the braiding of hair and the putting on of gold jewelry, or the clothing you wear, but let your adorning be the hidden person of the heart with the imperishable beauty of a gentle and quiet spirit." How many times do we see
ourselves in the mirror and make negative comments about our looks.
I'm not pretty or I'm too fat or I'm too overweight. These are few of the phrases that
first come to mind in most girls when they look at themselves in the mirror. Well, 90% of teenage girls do not like the way they look or appear. The reason for that is - in our society you get attention from people if you look attractive and stunning.

Some girls who are overweight would get negative comments from peers like- 'That girl is too ugly' or 'That girl looks like a bulldozer'. Fat is not something you have, it is something you are. We don't say "You have fat," we say, "You are fat." We identify with our bodies. So the teenager gets the message that this fatness is badness. Some of the teenagers who don't accept the way they look, try to change themselves by dieting which leads to illnesses and diseases like anorexia.

Dieting is the practice of ingesting food in a regulated fashion to achieve or maintain a controlled weight. In most cases the goal is weight loss in those who are overweight or obese, but some people these days start dieting because they want to change the way they appear to the society. But what really matters in life? An old proverb states, "Beauty is in the eye of the beholder." Something or someone is beautiful, depending on the perspective of the person looking in but the major thing that matters is the person good-looking from inside? Without a doubt inner beauty lasts forever whereas outer beauty fades. Anyone can fake the outside to make himself or herself look better and pretty but inner beauty can't be faked. For example you could be the most beautiful person in the world but if you have a horrible personality it just makes you ugly. Your body image is how you perceive, think and feel about your body but this may have no link at all on your actual appearance.

Here's a poem by my friend Conner on Inner Beauty

I don't care about your looks,
or the kind of clothes you wear.
I don't care about your make-up,
or the way you fix your hair.

What I care about is you,
and your beauty on the inside.
A beauty so amazing,
that it can never subside.

A beauty that brings me up,
when I'm falling down.
A beauty that makes me smile,
instead of frown.

What lies in you is rare,
yet so true.
A sense of comfort is felt,
when I spend time with you.

No emotion like the one I have,
when I hear the sweet sound of your voice.
No words to put my feelings into,
only pure rejoice.

A beautiful girl,
in each aspect of her life and soul.
A beautiful girl,
that completes me and makes me whole.

4 OUTER BEAUTY

What is outer beauty?

Outer beauty is a term that refers to the external qualities that pleases the intellect or moral sense. It involves physical care of the body. Other terms that mean the same as beauty include pulchritude and loveliness. We know it is greatly appreciated and very important for a lot of people. Many would argue that it is how you look and how other people react to your physical appearance that really matters. To look good is to feel good. But is it really that important and if so how do we reach outer beauty. Outer beauty is thought to be something that you are born with. It is either there or it isn't. Those attractive features that make people notice you in a crowd. A face, a figure, outer beauty is basically about flesh and bone. How good we look.

My Opinion On Outer Beauty

Okay, let's admit it. Most of us say that inner beauty is more important than outer beauty... blah, blah, blah.. Now, my question is, if so, then why are you still working on your outer beauty? I do admit that I'm one of those girls who spend time and money trying to be more beautiful - well, I do not spend a lot though. I do it because I want to be more presentable to other people, and I know that a lot of girls do things to make them look more beautiful for the same reason. I just cannot help it. I think it is the reason why still a lot of people spend money on cosmetics and beauty procedures. Even if they say that beauty comes from within and everything, they still want to look beautiful outside even more than they are inside. It's funny but it's true. When will we learn to "do as we say"? For me, it's really important to look good outside because that is the first thing people would see in you. And most people would like to know someone better if they are attracted first with how they look outside. I think that is why I value outer beauty so much. Whether we admit it or not, we always have the tendency to judge people and like people first on how they appear outside, right?

Attraction

Of course we feel physically drawn to certain physical features and forms, feeling attracted to a certain person. Some like it slim, other plus sized. Point is this attraction is highly individual. Like we argued about inner beauty, outer beauty is in the eye of the beholder.

The Perception of Outer Beauty

Every day we are exposed to a commercialized image on how the male and female body and look should be like. Posters of hair products where the posing model has "perfect" figure and hair or in TV-shows where actors and actresses look like Barbie and Ken dolls. This is the perception of outer beauty that we learn to yearn and strive to be. But it is not real outer beauty. Real outer beauty does not come in only one size and shape. Any shape and look is attractive. That is a fact!

You are beautiful

Your job is to find that person who can't stop looking at you, who finds you irresistible. Don't settle for anyone else just because you are comparing yourself with the image on the poster and on the TV-screen. That is one form of outer beauty but not necessarily yours.

Outer Beauty is Inner Beauty And It Does Matter

Remember outer beauty is a reflection of your inner beauty, your self-confidence and how you fell about the things you do. If you don't feel beautiful, you won't look beautiful. But if your confidence is up and you are feeling good about your thoughts, values and personality it will create an outer beauty that does not really have to do with shapes or forms.

Let's Sum It Up

Do you think of outer beauty as a surface aesthetic or represented only by what you can see or hear like looks, or do you think of outer beauty as the whole package both the outer shell and the inner person? Do you think of attraction as one sided or mutual? Are you talking about gravity or gravitas in attraction? There is a simple answer to this question, outer beauty is a subset of attraction. If attraction is something that attracts, and outer beauty is something that attracts, they are similar in that outer beauty is an attraction, but so is a waterslide. Attraction covers more than just sexuality or sensuality, but outer beauty is strictly an interpersonal attraction, strictly sensual or sexual. On the other hand I tend to think of attraction as "a force acting mutually between particles of matter, tending to draw them together, and resisting their separation" since that is really where the term has its start in science, I think of the romantic part of what that could mean. So attraction is some irresistible force between two people that draws them together and creates a bond. Attraction is a partnership, an unwritten unspoken agreement between two strangers to become friends, to become lovers. For me then outer beauty is an aesthetic quality that one can appreciate and that can encourage attraction but is not solely to attract. A person can find something or someone beautiful and stop there, no need to define the others relationship to that person. Lastly, attraction has a hazy higher level feeling that is almost mystical even ethereal, outer beauty it's actually almost entirely temporal and worldly.

5 MENTAL HEALTH

Mental health describes a level of psychological well- being, or an absence of a mental disorder. From the perspective of 'positive psychology' or 'holism', mental health may include an individual's ability to enjoy life, and create a balance between life activities and efforts to achieve psychological resilience. Mental health can also be defined as an expression of emotions, and as signifying a successful adaptation to a range of demands. The word' health organization defines mental health as "a state of well- being in which the individual realizes his or her own abilities, can cope with the normal stresses of life, can work productively and fruitfully, and is able to make a contribution to his or her community". It was previously stated that there was no "official" definition of mental health. Cultural differences, subjective assessments, and competing professional theories all affect how "mental health" is defined. There are different types of mental health problems, some of which are common, such as depression and anxiety disorders, and some not so common, such as schizophrenia and bipolar disorder. Most recently, the field of global mental health has emerged, which has been defined as 'the area of study, research and practice that places a priority on improving mental health and achieving equity in mental health for all people worldwide. So in order to be able to love yourself and feel beautiful, your mental health must be stable.

According to the World Health Organization in 2004, depression is the leading cause of disability in the United States of America for individuals ages 15 to 44. Absence from work in the U.S. due to depression is estimated to be in excess of $31 billion per year. Depression frequently co-occurs with a variety of medical illnesses such as heart disease, cancer, and chronic pain and is associated with poorer health status and prognosis. Each year, roughly 30,000 Americans take their lives, while hundreds of thousands make suicide attempts (center for disease control and prevention). In 2004, suicide was the 11th leading -case of death in the United States of America (centers for disease control and prevention), third among individuals ages 15–24. Despite the increasingly availability of effectual depression treatment, the level of unmet need for treatment remains high. Being mentally and emotionally healthy does not preclude the experiences of life which we cannot control. As humans we are going to face emotions and events that are a part of life. According to Smith and Segal, "People who are emotionally and mentally healthy have the tools for coping with difficult situations and maintaining a positive outlook in which they also remain focused, flexible, and creative in bad times as well as good" (2011). In order to improve your emotional mental health, the root of the issue has to be resolved.

"Prevention emphasizes the avoidance of risk factors; promotion aims to enhance an individual's ability to achieve a positive sense of self -esteem, mastery, well-being, and social inclusion" (power, 2010). It is very important to improve your emotional mental health by surrounding yourself with positive relationships. We as humans, feed off companionships and interaction with other people. Another way to improve your emotional mental health is participating in activities that can allow you to relax and take time for yourself. Yoga is a great example of an activity that calms your entire body and nerves. According to a study on well-being by Richards, Campania and Muse-Burke, "mindfulness is considered to be a purposeful state, it may be that those who practice it believe in its importance and value being mindful, so that valuing of self-care activities may influence the intentional component of mindfulness" Increased awareness of mental processes can influence emotional behavior and mental health. A 2011 study incorporating three types of meditative practice (concentration meditation, mindfulness meditation and compassion toward others) revealed that meditation provides an enhanced ability to recognize emotions in others and their own emotional patterns, so they could better resolve difficult problems in their relationships.

I like to think of mental health as being sane or content with yourself and your surroundings. A sense of being at peace or "one with nature". Being in good physical shape and having proper nutrition is very important, however, many forget about mental health. Sometimes people hook their self-worth on their appearance, tying beauty to their perception of themselves, says Heather Patrick, researcher at the National Institutes of Health. "We compare how we think we look to how other people look, and we make a decision about whether we're much better or much worse," she said. That comparison can have negative or positive emotional and psychological consequences. There's scientific evidence to suggest that ideas about the importance of one's own beauty get formulated in childhood, she said. Parents give a certain level of praise to their children for their appearance, vs. the amount of effort they put into tasks and the activities they're good at. Little girls in child beauty contests, for instance, receive the feedback that their appearance is highly valued. That sets the stage for people to think about themselves in terms of appearance or abilities. When it comes to assessing beauty, many people are their own worst critics. Sometimes there's a particular body part that becomes a focus of self-loathing. of ourselves in the same way that we filter judgments of others."

When taken to the extreme, obsession over a particular aspect of one's appearance has a psychiatric diagnosis: body dysmorphic disorder. It's the reason some people get dozens of plastic surgeries, but are never satisfied with the outcomes. On the flip side, you can view your body as a source of power -- for instance, after running a first 5 kilometer race or even marathon, some people feel proud of what their bodies can do. Regardless of culture, there appear to be certain patterns of brain activity associated with viewing something you find beautiful. Neuro-esthetic research has found that the only factor common to all that people find beautiful in art and music is activity in the brain's medial orbital frontal cortex, part of the reward and pleasure center of the brain. There are cultural trends in what in art and music people find beautiful for instance, there's a Japanese preference for asymmetry, compared to a Western ideal of symmetry. This does not apply to faces, however, as it seems that universally people prefer symmetrical faces. It's also not well understood why people adapt to certain objects of beauty after many exposures, but not others. For instance, you might be bored of a pop song after a few listens, but listen to an opera dozens of times, over a period of years, and still feel emotional about it. Perhaps there's a painting that you've always admired, where another painting loses its splendor after a few viewings. That makes sense, since we see every single blemish in ourselves, whereas there are plenty of people we consider beautiful to whom we don't get close enough to examine all the little flaws. Perception of beauty may weaken when we do start to recognize those defects. Imaging of the brain has been done with facial beauty as well. A recent study in neuro-image found that self-evaluation of one's own facial attractiveness may be a result of that person's self-esteem which are based on common patterns of brain activity.

6 LOVE YOUR HAIR

As women we take great pride in our grooming and besides our skin and physique, one of our most important beauty parts is our hair. We should care for our hair and make sure that it is healthy and shiny. So I have researched and also shared with you some of my hair care secrets. I think that you'll enjoy this do it yourself process. After all it's all part of loving ourselves.

Make an all-natural remedy designed especially for your hair type.

Homemade Hair Treatments

Eggs, yogurt and honey are, at first glance, all components of a tasty breakfast, but they also happen to be hair treatment ingredients, and affordable, all-natural ones at that. And they're not the only ones. Did you know, for instance, that the oils in avocados more closely resemble our own skin's oils than any product in the beauty aisle does? Or that the mild acidity in lemon is an effective and gentler alternative to chemical-laden products? Next time your locks need a lift, save money by using one of these kitchen fixes.

For All Hair Types

The egg yolk, rich in fats and proteins, is naturally moisturizing, while the white, which contains bacteria-eating enzymes, removes unwanted oils, she explains.

To Use: For normal hair, use the entire egg to condition hair; use egg whites only to treat oily hair; use egg yolks only to moisturize dry, brittle hair. Use 1/2 cup of whichever egg mixture is appropriate for you and apply to clean, damp hair. If there isn't enough egg to coat scalp and hair, use more as needed. Leave on for 20 minutes, rinse with cool water (to prevent egg from "cooking") and shampoo hair. Whole egg and yolks-only treatments can be applied once a month; whites-only treatment can be applied every two weeks.

For Dull Hair

Styling products (as well as air pollution) can leave a film that both saps moisture and dulls shine but dairy products like sour cream and plain yogurt can help reverse this damage..

To Use: Massage 1/2 cup sour cream or plain yogurt into damp hair and let sit for 20 minutes. Rinse with warm water, followed by cool water, then shampoo hair as you normally would. Treatment can be applied every other week.

For Itchy Scalp

To fight flakes brought on by poor diet, stress and climate, among other factors, try a lemon juice and olive oil mixture in your hair. "The acidity in lemon juice helps rid your scalp of any loose, dry flakes of skin, while the olive oil moisturizes the [newly exposed] skin on your head".
To Use: Mix 2 tablespoons fresh lemon juice, 2 tablespoons olive oil and 2 tablespoons water, and massage into damp scalp. Let mixture sit for 20 minutes, then rinse and shampoo hair. Treatment can be applied every other week.

For Limp or Fine Hair

To add body to hair, reach for an unlikely beauty beverage: beer! The fermented drink contains generous supplies of yeast, which works to plump tired tresses.
To Use: Mix 1/2 cup flat beer (pour beer into a container and let it sit out for a couple of hours to deplete carbonation) with 1 tablespoon light oil (sunflower or canola) and a raw egg. Apply to clean, damp hair, let sit for 15 minutes, then rinse with cool water. Or add flat beer only to a spray bottle and spritz onto dry hair. "When the liquid evaporates, the remaining protein residue (from the wheat, malt or hops) continues to strengthen and structure hair,". Treatments can be applied every other week.

For Dry or Sun-Damaged Hair

Whatever your hair-dehydrating demon, hard water, sun overexposure, your trusty flat iron nature's sweetener can help. "Honey is a natural humectant, which means it attracts and locks in moisture,".

To Use: Massage approximately 1/2 cup honey into clean, damp hair, let sit for 20 minutes, then rinse with warm water. You can also add 1 to 2 tablespoons olive oil to loosen the honey for easier application. For extremely sun-damaged hair, trying mixing honey with 1 to 2 tablespoons of a protein-rich ingredient, like avocado or egg yolk, which will help replenish the keratin protein bonds that UV rays attack. Treatment can be applied once a month.

For Oily or Greasy Hair

"Used properly, (cornmeal or cornstarch) is an inexpensive way to remove oil and grease,".

To Use: Pour 1 tablespoon cornmeal or cornstarch into an empty salt or pepper shaker and sprinkle onto dry hair and scalp until you've used it all. After 10 minutes, use a paddle hairbrush to completely brush it out. Treatment can be applied every other day.

For Frizzy Hair

Home beauty experts swear by avocado and not just to repair damaged hair. Its oils (which are light and moist like our own natural skin secretions) and proteins boast the best combination of nutrients for smoothing and weighing down unruly hair, explains Cox.

To Use: Mash up half an avocado and massage into clean, damp hair. Let sit for 15 minutes before rinsing with water. Amp up moisturizing power by combining mashed avocado with 1 to 2 tablespoons of a hydrating ingredient, like sour cream, egg yolks or mayonnaise. Treatment can be applied every two weeks.

For Residue-Ridden Hair

"Nothing eats through product buildup like baking soda," Cox says. Sodium bicarbonate essentially breaks down anything acidic.

To Use: Mix 1 to 2 tablespoons baking soda with small amounts of water until a thick paste forms. Massage into damp hair and let sit for 15 minutes. Rinse with water, then shampoo hair. Treatment can be applied every two weeks.

Hair Loss:

One can suffer from hair loss at any age
The condition generally results in a receding hair line

Symptoms to look for:
Hair fall
Development of bald patches
Thinning of hair in women
Causes:

Stress

Weakness

Anemia

Lack of proper nutrition

Vitamin B6 and folic acid deficiency

Unclean scalp, which blocks and weakens the hair pores

Hereditary factors

Natural home remedy using Indian gooseberry and lemon juice:

1. Cut and de-seed an Indian gooseberry
2. Crush the cut gooseberry to paste
3. Press this paste on a sieve and extract its juice
4. Add 3 tbsp lemon juice to this juice
5. Mix well
6. Apply this on the scalp
7. Leave it for 30 min
8. Wash off with normal water

Natural home remedy using curry leaves, lemon peel, soap nut, fenugreek seeds and green gram:

1. Take 15-20 curry leaves
2. Add 1 lemon peel
3. Add 3 tbsp soap nut powder
4. Add 2 tbsp fenugreek seeds
5. Add 2 tbsp green gram
6. Grind the mixture and store in a clean, glass bottle
7. Use this mixture as a shampoo

Natural home remedy using margosa leaves:

1. Boil handful of crushed margosa leaves in 4 cups of water
2. Cool and filter the liquid
3. Use this decoction to rinse your hair

Premature Greying of Hair:

Premature greying is when hair loses its natural pigmentation at an early age.

Causes:

Lack of nutrition to the scalp due to improper diet

Stress

Deficiency in vitamins like:

Iron
Copper
Iodine
Vitamin B
Not cleaning the scalp regularly
Using very hot water while washing hair
Excessive blow drying
Regular usage of hair dyes
Hereditary condition

Natural home remedy using Indian gooseberries:

1. Cut, deseed and crush 4-5 Indian gooseberries to a paste
2. Apply this paste on the scalp
3. Leave it for 15-20 min
4. Wash hair with normal water

Natural home remedy using curry leaves and coconut oil:

1. Take 7-8 crushed curry leaves
2. Add 3 tbsp of coconut oil
3. Heat this mixture for 5-7 min
4. Strain the mixture
5. Massage on scalp when lukewarm

Natural home remedy using lemon juice and almond oil:

1. Take 1 tsp of lemon juice
2. Add 2 tsp of almond oil
3. Mix well
4. Massage on the scalp
Tips:
 Massage scalp regularly with warm mustard or coconut oil to prevent premature greying

Facial Hair:

Facial hair is a natural phenomenon
But, having excess hair can be embarrassing, especially for women
Shaving facial hair is not advisable
Waxing is popular but is not advisable for women with sensitive skin
Plucking is a painful and time consuming method
Causes:
Hormonal imbalance
Irregular menstrual cycle
Certain medicines
Post-pregnancy hormonal changes

Natural home remedy using chickpea flour, milk, turmeric powder and fresh cream:

1. Take ½ bowl of chickpea flour
2. Add ½ cup milk
3. Add 1 tsp turmeric powder
4. Add 1 tsp fresh cream
5. Mix well
6. Apply and massage on the face, covering all hair
7. Leave it for 25 min and let the paste dry
8. Remove the dried paste by rubbing palms in direction opposite the hair growth.

Natural alternatives instead of using shampoo:

Frizzy Hair – (A natural replacement to shampoo)
But, without a doubt, the best way to treat frizzy hair is by ditching the shampoo completely. It's not always the right thing for straight, fine hair as it's typically suggested, but it's worth a try no matter your hair type.

How to go without shampoo:

Wash your scalp well with a solution of baking soda and water.
Rinse your hair well.
Finish by rinsing your ends with a solution of diluted apple cider vinegar.

Dandruff – Coconut Oil

To be completely honest, I haven't ever had a problem with dandruff (just product build-up back in the day), but I have lived with people who have the sneaky white stuff every once in a while, and after trying many remedies, I can safely say the answer is: Coconut oil. It has worked every single time in one or two treatments.
The key is to get virgin coconut oil that's been cold pressed – it's going to have all the active moisturizers and antibacterial properties that you need to quickly and efficiently cure yourself or someone you love (who probably wears a lot of hats). Guess what else? This is a stellar treatment for cradle cap, too. Yay babies!
(If you want to make it extra potent for adults, add in 5-7 drops of tea tree oil to your coconut oil.)

How to treat dandruff with coconut oil:

Before showering, massage 3-5 Tablespoons of coconut oil directly onto the scalp. Rub it all in there good.
Leave this on for at least an hour.
Shampoo as normal (or sort of shampoo as normal). There should be no need to use conditioner a coconut oil hair mask is a fantastic pre-conditioner.

Do this treatment every day up to five to seven days before giving up! And if you've forgotten, there are tons of other things you can do with coconut oil

For Longer Eyelashes

Petroleum Jelly
This inexpensive product, which has emollient and protective effects, is a mainstay of home remedies to increase eyelash length. First remove any eyeliner, eye shadow or mascara with a cotton ball, then apply petroleum jelly with a new mascara wand, or one that you have first cleaned well to remove any trace of the original product. I recommend sleeping with the petroleum jelly on your eyelashes, but washing it off in the morning before you go about your day. For best results, repeat the treatment three times a week.

Green Tea

Natural Home Remedies recommends applying cool, unsweetened green tea to your lashes with a cotton ball to take advantage of green tea beneficial properties. According to Whole Foods, green tea is rich in flavonoids, including epigallocatechin-3 gallate, which has potent antioxidant and health-supportive effects. As with all home remedies for eyelash growth, take care not to get the liquid into your eye, and rinse well with cool water if you do.

Olive Oil

I suggest that you use olive oil to help protect, condition and lengthen eyelashes. Apply at bedtime with a clean mascara brush. Keep the oil on overnight, then remove it in the morning with a gentle eye makeup remover, the olive oil can attract dirt and dust to your lashes.
Brushing and Caring For Eyelashes
To stimulate growth and promote healthy lashes, I advise that you use a commercial professional eyelash brush to groom lashes twice a day. As with brushing your hair, this can help distribute natural oils along the length of your lashes. To avoid stress on your lashes and eye area, always remove eye makeup before going to bed. International beauty also cautions against wearing mascara for prolonged periods of time.

Lemon Olive Oil

Natural Home Remedies suggests enhancing the healthful properties of olive oil by soaking a lemon peel in a jar of oil for several days, then carefully applying the mixture to your lashes. Lemon is a mild natural antiseptic and antimicrobial agent, and may help promote healthier lashes.

Proper Diet

You can enrich your diet to make sure you are getting the right nutrients and vitamins to promote eyelash growth. Eyelashes are made of keratin, a type of protein, and can benefit from a diet that includes high-protein foods like meat, fish, chicken, soy and tofu. Vitamin A, essential to lash growth, is found in eggs, fish oil, and red, yellow and orange fruits, while citrus fruits, potatoes and tomatoes are rich in vitamin C, a potent antioxidant. Calcium, also essential for lashes, is found in milk, as well as in dark green leafy vegetables.

Eyelid Massage

Massaging your eyelids gently can increase blood flow and may stimulate growth of lashes, according to Grow Eyelashes. After washing your hands well, use the pads of your fingers to massage along your lids and lash line.

7 LIVING IN YOUR SKIN

You may be surprised to learn your skin is actually your body's largest organ. Not only is it the largest organ accounting for approximately 16% of body weight, but it is also our protective armor. Good health often is reflected in an attractive, youthful appearance and so it is vitally important we look after this 'organ.' Skin is truly amazing, one of the most complex organs in the body.

Skin – The Facts

Human skin comprises an outer layer known as the epidermis, a middle layer of tissue called the dermis and underlying these is the subcutaneous layer that includes sebaceous and sweat glands, blood vessels, sense organs and nerves. Skin is predominantly made up of collagen. Collagen, important for maintaining healthy skin, is a natural protein that provides 'building blocks' supporting the growth of new cells by binding them together within the skin. Skin texture and natural moisture content are different around the eyes, lips, neck and cleavage or chest. It's a fact that everyone, women and men alike, wants to remain as young and fresh looking for as long as possible.

Skin Aging

 It's a fact that everyone, women and men alike, wants to remain as young and fresh looking for as long as possible. People in their twenties tend to be more cautious in their skincare regime and by the late thirties and beyond it's all about maintenance. As we age the natural cellular activity of the skin slows gradually causing skin to lose its ability to retain moisture and protein resulting in loss of tautness and tone. This causes the appearance of fine lines and wrinkles. From the age of twenty five years onwards, levels of collagen naturally diminish over time approximately by as much as 1.5% per year. Helping the skin to replace this lost collagen can help to improve the elasticity of the skin and naturally help to reduce the appearance of fine lines and wrinkles. The eyes, mouth, neck, cleavage or chest are more vulnerable to skin ageing and have a tendency to be over-looked in the daily skincare routine. Daily cleansing and toning, as well as eating a healthy, nutrient-packed diet, keeping yourself well hydrated and getting sufficient exercise and sleep are important to help maintain skin health.

Following are some solutions to common issues with our skin:

Beauty- Puffy Eyes – Green Tea Ice Cubes

I've needed this remedy quite a few times lately, what with allergies and other puffy-eyed demons rearing their heads. This is particularly nice, because you can freeze up a whole batch of these and use them whenever you need them – for as long as you need them (they last forever in the freezer).
Just pop them out of the ice cube trays once they're frozen and keep them in a small lidded jar or bag in your freezer until the morning they'll come in handy.

How to make green tea ice cubes:

Brew one or two strong (very strong) cups of green tea.
Leave the leaves in if you're making it with loose-leaf tea, or strain (or get rid of your tea bags) if not.
Wait 30 minutes for the tea to cool.
Pour in ice cube tray(s) and freeze.
Green tea isn't just great for puffy eyes, but it's a wonder for acne and oily skin, as well – so don't be afraid to rub that ice cube over your whole face if you want – especially if that whole face is puffy.

Massage the skin with aromatherapy

Aging and weight-loss decrease the skins elasticity and firmness due to the loss and breakdown of collagen in the dermal layer of your skin and as a result the skin can become loose and thin.

Aromatherapy is the natural way to help tighten the skin without chemicals or invasive treatment. The massage will help to tone the muscles, keep muscles supple and aid absorption of the aromatherapy oil.

Some of the best aromatherapy essential oils for firming and toning the skin is rosemary (stimulating, firming oil) frankincense (delay signs of ageing) and neroli (increase circulation and moisturising). Other powerful essentials oils good for toning the skin include jasmine, lavender, rose, sandalwood, myrrh, patchouli, geranium and rose.

Add a couple of aromatherapy drops to 2 tablespoons of carrier oil such as carrot oil (mix with 1 tablespoons of another carrier) jojoba, avocado oil or a vitamin E cream before the massage. Apply the cream or oil to the area.

Apply in a slow upward movement always working towards the heart, this will help increase the circulation to the muscles and skin. Knead into the area by wringing the skin between cupped hands. Finish the massage with a slow, upward movement.

Apply the oil or cream morning and night.

Chapped Lips – Baking Soda Exfoliation and Cocoa Butter

I hesitated to put this in here, because we're about to start a new challenge where we'll all be getting ready for winter with different wintertime/cold/flu remedies to have on hand.
So consider this a tiny preview of what's to come – during the "winter skin" day.

Fix those chapped lips:

 In a small bowl, combine baking soda and milk or sour cream until you have a thick paste.
 Lightly (very lightly) scrub your dry lips with this paste in a circular motion for 2-3 minutes.
 Rinse well with water.

 Finish by slathering on cocoa butter (or your favorite natural lip balm – I just prefer to use a thick coating of cocoa butter).
This may not cure the chapped lips immediately, but it will get you moving in the right direction. Just remember to continue to slather on cocoa butter or lip balm every few hours. And don't do the exfoliation if your lips are bleeding. Ouch! Let them heal first, and then go for it.

Monster Pimples – Lavender Essential Oil and Clay

This is one of those remedies that may or may not work for you (I've heard varying results).

All you need is a little bit of cosmetic clay (which you can find at Mountain Rose Herbs or any natural food store), lavender essential oil, and a few drops of water.

Get rid of that giant pimple like this:

In a small bowl or the palm of your hand, pour about 1/2 tsp of clay.

Drop in 2-3 drops of lavender essential oil (or you could use tea tree or peppermint if that's what you have on hand).

Pour in a teeny tiny bit of water and smash the clay around until everything is combined and the clay is pasty (adding more water if necessary – but be careful, a little goes a long way).

Dab your tiny clay mask onto the pimple area.

Leave this on for at least an hour or you can also leave it on overnight.

Apple Cider Vinegar

Everyone knows that vinegar enhances the flavor of foods and cleans windows like no other. But, did you know that apple cider vinegar is an excellent health and beauty aid? You might want to want to check and possibly replenish your supply of apple cider vinegar because it's good for so many things. It amazing but be sure to only use organic apple cider vinegar. I swear by Bragg's organic apple cider vinegar. It's the best gift that I have ever given to myself. Seriously you guys, it's just good for so many things, it's brilliant.

Here are just some of the many things you can use vinegar to treat your skin:

Relieve a sun burn by rubbing vinegar on your skin.

-Use as a deodorant, just wipe your arm pits with a cloth moistened in vinegar and it will help you smell fresh for hours. If stinky feet are a problem for you soak your feet every night for 10 minutes or more in a solution of 1 ounce of vinegar in a gallon of water.

- You can treat the varicose veins in your legs by wrapping your legs with a cloth dampened with apple cider vinegar. To get the best possible results drink a glass of warm water with 1 to 2 teaspoons of apple cider vinegar after each treatment.

- You can treat the varicose veins in your legs by wrapping your legs with a cloth dampened with apple cider vinegar. To get the best possible results drink a glass of warm water with 1 to 2 teaspoons of apple cider vinegar after each treatment.

- Fade age or liver spots by wiping every day with a mixture of 2 teaspoons vinegar and 1 teaspoon onion juice.

-.To help prevent and eliminate facial blemishes steam clean your face by draping a towel over your head and placing your face over a steaming pan of ¼ cup vinegar and 1 quart of water. Please be really careful when doing this, steam can cause really bad burns. Once your pores are open, wipe apple cider vinegar over your face with a cotton ball to clean and loosen dirt and oil then splash your face with a half and half mix of cold water and cool vinegar to close.

-Help out your nail polish by cleaning your nails with vinegar before applying the polish. This will help the polish to last longer your pores.

- Relieve chapped hands by applying apple cider vinegar several times a day.

- If corn's are a problem for you try soaking a slice of onion in vinegar and bind it to the corn overnight or just apply a drop of vinegar to the corn every night.

- If poison ivy is a problem for you try daubing equal parts of apple cider vinegar and water to the rash and let it dry.

-Apply vinegar to a cold sore to help it heal quickly and relived the pain and discomfort.

Keratosis Polaris (Or Those Bumps On Your Upper Arms) – ACV (apple cider vinegar) and Sugar Scrub

These funny chicken bumps on your upper arms are common, so don't feel too bad. In fact, this is a very common situation.
 (And, trust me, I actually have a friend who has tried dozens of things and this was the most magical).

Wash with apple cider vinegar and then using a gentle sugar scrub afterward. It will take two or three times of doing this to see any difference, but once you see improvement it will vanish almost immediately.

 Here's how to have no more chicken arms!

1. In the shower, wash your upper arms with apple cider vinegar (you can dilute it or just use a teaspoon on a wet washcloth).
 Rinse your arms with water.

2. Finish with a very gentle sugar scrub using 1/2 c. sugar with 1/2 c. coconut oil or grape seed oil mixed in (which you can put in a jar and leave in your bathroom at all times if desired).

3. After massaging gently for a minute or two, rinse this off and enjoy your arms – finally!

Aging With Beauty and Grace

Wrinkles:

Skin loses its elasticity with age
Wrinkles are creases caused in skin when it thins and sags due to old age.
Wrinkles first appear near the eye and with age, they appear on cheeks, lips, neck and hand .
Causes:
Rough environmental conditions can cause premature wrinkles. Chemicals present in the smoke can destroy skin cells.

Natural home remedy using egg whites:

1. Egg whites contain vitamins, which help tighten skin
2. Apply egg whites on wrinkle prone areas
3. Leave for 20 min
4. Wash with lukewarm water

Natural home remedy using avocado, fresh cream, flaxseeds and honey:

1. Crush and make paste of ½ an avocado
2. Add 2 tbsp of fresh cream
3. Add 2 tsp of flaxseeds
4. Add 1 tbsp of honey
5. Mix well
6. Apply on the skin and leave it for 1 hour
7. Wash with cold water
8. This mixture is a natural moisturizer

Natural home remedy using papaya and banana:

This remedy workswonders
1. Blend papaya and banana together
2. Apply on the skin
3. Leave it for 20 min
4. Wash it off with lukewarm water
Papaya has chemicals, which remove dead skin cells. Banana provides necessary nutrients for healthy skin.

Chia Seeds
I use chia seed on my face. Here's how:

Chia: Rise and Shine
They are crazy high in alpha-lipoic acids. Better known as ALA. Better known as that-ingredient-that-makes-skin-cream-cost-a-bajillion-dollars. Alpha-lipoic acid is said to help with cell function, promote radiance in the skin, help diminish fine lines, and aid in antioxidant effectiveness. So it makes sense that these little seeds would be a perfect morning facial scrub. And, yes it diminishes fine lines and make your skin feel very soft and clear all day long. Here's how I (and how you, too, can) incorporate chia seeds into a morning ritual – by putting them on your face! Then, I stir it up again and pour just a small amount (maybe 1 Tbsp) of the mixture into my hands and start scrubbing/rubbing my face with it. Without rinsing (yet), I drink the "chia seed honey water" and let the mixture on my face chill out for a while. Five to ten minutes, tops. Then, I rinse. And enjoy a soft face. Lovely. Here's the cool part. You don't have to use water. I just like it for its simplicity. You could also use full-fat milk or coconut milk (great for dry or aging skin), almond milk, or even a fresh-pressed apple juice if you'd like (extra exfoliating, with the acids in the apple). It is an awesome way to start the day. For your face. By the way, you can get chia seeds almost anywhere these days. All major health food stores sell them. Whole Foods has excellent prices on organic chia, and you'll find them in any natural foods store as well.

The Power Raw Garlic

Garlic has many beauty and healing uses due to its antiviral, antibacterial, antifungal, and antioxidant, antiseptic and anti - aging properties.

How garlic can be used for clearing skin of acne?

Squeeze out juice of one garlic, mix with a small amount of apple cider vinegar and apply 2 times a day to pimples and acne. Garlic will repair skin, protect it from further damage and will help to get rid of infection. It is able to heal old acne scars and can heal burns. To get rid of odor, garlic clove can be placed into the milk before squeezing the juice.
To keep skin bright and acne - free, it is helpful to add chopped garlic to food. Another way to use garlic is to put it in blender with juice or add to yogurts to soften its taste.

Garlic is powerful when is used against athlete's foot. Crushed garlic is simply applied to the affected area till the symptoms vanish. Garlic is effective against warts: small piece of garlic is secured with a band- aid at night; it will take about a week of applications to kill the wart. The way to know that garlic's job is finished, is when there is no burning sensation left after new application.

Ginger's Powerful Rejuvenation

First, it must be pointed out that because we're working with fresh ginger, these things aren't going to stay preserved for as long as you'd probably hope. In fact, you should use your ginger immediately.

Here's a great ginger tip:

To peel ginger, just use the side of a spoon. This is a pretty well-known tip, but it must be mentioned. You don't need a fancy peeler to peel the skin from the ginger – in fact, I often feel that my peeler is too thorough when I use it on ginger. Just tilt your spoon to the side and use the edge to scrape down the ginger. The top layer should peel off easily and quickly.

Rejuvenating Ginger-Lemon Body Scrub(reduces cellulite)

One of ginger's most notable qualities is its invigorating, fresh, and spicy feeling. Add it with a bit of lemon zest in a sugar scrub, and you have a body scrub that will warm you up and wake you up at the same time.

And here's a secret for you: Ginger is highly-regarded as one of nature's best cellulite reducers, so if you do this regularly, you may see a difference in the bumps!

Fresh Ginger-Lemon Body Scrub

1/2 c. organic sugar
1/4 c. olive oil
2 tsp freshly grated, peeled ginger
Zest from one organic lemon
Combine all ingredients in a small bowl. Stir well. In the shower or bath,
scrub your body lightly with the mixture and rinse well. This should keep in
the refrigerator (if necessary) for up to a week. But I highly recommend you
use it immediately.

Fresh Ginger for Hypo-pigmented Scars (or White Scars)

Hypo-pigmented scars or skin has lost its pigmentation and is either white or
a much lighter color than your actual skin tone. Incredibly enough, ginger will
fix this issue.
I first read about this phenomenon in one of my natural beauty books, but I
took to the internet to find out if anyone had any practical experience with
ginger actually helping to return the skin to its natural color.
And yes. Yes, there is plentiful anecdotal evidence that ginger actually
significantly reduces the appearance of hypo-pigmented skin.

In the meantime, here's how you do it: Each day (or even twice a day) cut a
very small sliver of fresh ginger and dab it on the hypo-pigmented areas.
Don't wash it off. Just leave the juice there. According to the forums I've
read, most people see a slight improvement within a week or two, and within
a few months, their scars are nearly completely back to normal color. The
important thing is, do this every day.

How to Whiten Skin With Natural Products

Age spots, acne scars and other blemishes often keep you from having a good complexion. There are hundreds of formulas and products on the shelves that promise to give the skin an even and brighter appearance. Before spending money on products full of questionable ingredients, consider trying natural remedies and products to whiten and brighten the skin.

Instructions

1. Exfoliate the skin regularly. Exfoliation removes dead skin cells and gives the skin a brighter appearance. Products applied to the face can be absorbed more effectively by the skin as a result. A natural scrub can be made by mixing brown sugar with lemon juice, which is a natural skin whitener, and olive oil. Apply the scrub to damp skin and rub in gently. Rinse your face thoroughly. This scrub can be done once a week or as needed.

2. Apply a brightening mask to the skin weekly. Ingredients like papaya will lighten the skin. Egg whites will tighten the skin, and yogurt and honey will moisturize it. You can make a mask by mixing all of these ingredients together until you have a thick, creamy consistency. Apply the mask to the face and leave on for about 10 minutes. Use cool water to remove the mask.

3. Invest in a skin cream or skin serum that contains kojic acid. Kojic acid is considered a safer skin-whitening alternative to hydroquinone, according to the Health Life Journal website. Apply according to directions.

4. Try soaps with natural whitening ingredients like papaya and black licorice. A few companies sell whitening soaps with these as the main ingredients.

5. Keep skin moisturized. Some skin-whitening ingredients, though natural, can be drying. Vitamin E oil and aloe vera are excellent for moisturizing the skin.

6. Research natural sunscreens and choose one according to your skin type and level of sun protection you need. There are many on the market.

Nails

Homemade nail polish removers: New coat: One of the simple tips to remove nail polish is by applying a new coat of the nail paint and then immediately rub the nail on a cotton ball. This removes the nail paint naturally!

Vinegar: Soak a cotton ball in vinegar and rub on the nails. You can add lemon or orange juice in it and use as a homemade nail polish remover. Vinegar takes time to soften the nail polish so keep rubbing on the nails.
Alcohol: Rubbing alcohol is a simple homemade nail polish remover alternative. Soak a cotton ball in alcohol and rub on the nails. It may take few attempts to remove the nail polish completely.
Lemon: This is another natural ingredient to remove nail polish. Just rub a slice of lemon on the nails and remove the nail paint. It is also a natural manicure recipe. For best results, soak the nails in warm soapy water for 3-6 minutes to soften the nail polish. Then rub a lemon slice as a nail polish remover alternative. These are few homemade nail polish remover alternatives.

Blemishes:

A blemish is a discolored or a marked area on the skin.
Causes:

Marks may develop on skin due to skin conditions like boils, pimples or acne. Other causes include, skin injuries, age, sun spots, freckles and moles.

Natural home remedy using almonds and milk:

1. Soak 7-8 almonds in water for 12 hours
2. Peel and crush them
3. Add a little milk to make a paste
4. Apply on blemishes
5. Leave it overnight
6. Wash with cold water in the morning
7. Do this for at least 2 weeks

Natural home remedy using potato:

1. Take a potato slice
2. Rub on the affected area for 10 min
3. Do this 2-3 times a day

Natural home remedy using mint leaves:

1. Crush some mint leaves into a fine paste
2. Apply this paste on the blemishes
3. Leave it for 20 min
4. Wash it off with cold water

Stretch Marks:

Stretch marks usually appear on:
Abdomen, Back, Waist, Arms, Hips, Breast, Lower back and Legs.

Symptoms to look for:

Stretch marks are thick red or purple lines on the skin
 Over time, these lines fade to white or silver in color
Causes:

Skin is made up of elastin, which is a soft elastic tissue. It makes the skin soft, supple and stretchable. Over-stretching of skin damages elastin resulting in stretch marks. Sudden weight change. Rapid body growth during teenage pregnancy.

Natural home remedy using apricots:

1. Cut and remove seeds of 2-3 apricots
2. Crush them to paste
3. Apply this paste on the marks
4. Leave it for 20 min
5. Wash it off with lukewarm water
6. Repeat this regularly for 1 month

Natural home remedy using aloe vera:

1. Aloe vera has plant collagen which repairs the skin.
2. Remove the thorns and outer skin of a few aloe vera leaves
3. Extract the gel from inside
4. Apply this gel on the stretch marks
5. Leave it for 2 hr
6. Wash it off with normal water

Natural home remedy using lavender oil, chamomile oil and almond oil:

1. Take ½ tsp lavender oil
2. Add ½ tsp chamomile oil
3. Add 2 tsp almond oil
4. Mix well
5. Apply on the stretch marks

Apply petroleum jelly on the abdomen during pregnancy. Please Do Not do this without consulting your doctor.

8 PEARLY WHITES

Preserving our teeth is very important. For all human beings this is our pride and beauty as well. Having a mouth full of straight, egg-shell white teeth is essential when taking into consideration our beauty attributes as well a good hygiene. The mouth is the window to your health. So off course we all know that an apple a day keeps the doctor away. Also brushing your teeth after each meal is very important. Laying off the sweets, avoid cavities. Oh and here's a tip I got off one of my ex- boyfriend's, who happens to be a dentist; If you've had a glass of wine or any type of alcohol, give yourself at least forty- five minutes to an hour before brushing your teeth. If you brush your teeth right after drinking alcohol, they will wither away because of the acid from the alcohol which makes your teeth more sensitive and soft than ever.

Natural beauty secrets for teeth

If you have a toothache tea tree oil then just apply to the tooth.

Teeth Whitening

Strawberries- Strawberries may help whiten teeth because they contain an enzyme called malic acid, which can be found in some whitening toothpastes, celebrity beauty expert and author of "Hollywood Beauty Secrets: Remedies to the Rescue. You can mash up strawberry or just rub it on your teeth, cut in half. Leave the juice on your teeth for one minute and then rinse with water. The fiber in strawberries also behaves as a natural cleaner by removing bacteria from the teeth and mouth.

Apples, **Celery And Carrots**- These fruits and veggies act like natural stain removers. The reason: They increase saliva production, which is the body's built-in cleaning agent. "It may sound hard to believe, but some people swear that rubbing raw carrot sticks on your teeth will make them look brighter," said Gross. The added bonus: "These foods are high in vitamin C, which prevents gum disease and gingivitis and kills odor-causing bacteria.

Citrus Fruit- Citrus fruit, such as oranges and pineapples, also cause the mouth to produce more saliva, which help clean the teeth and whiten your smile, said Apa. Lemons, in particular, are particularly good for teeth whitening. "Just as they naturally 'bleach' your hair, lemons will lighten and brighten your teeth. It is suggested rinsing with half water, half lemon juice once or twice a week.
However, do not rinse with this concoction more than two times a week and do not rinse with straight lemon juice. "Overdoing it would be too acidic, which can be damaging to the teeth."

Yogurt, Milk And Cheese- "Dairy products have lactic acid, which decreases gum disease and maintains development and maintenance of teeth," said Apa. "Even the milk in coffee counts -- and it has the added benefit of [decreasing] coffee's staining ability." Along with protecting and strengthening the enamel, hard cheeses, like cheddar, are more effective at cleaning and whitening the teeth than softer cheeses, since hard cheese helps remove other food particles. "And keep in mind that dairy products and foods fortified with calcium and vitamin D are important not only for healthy teeth but your jawbone, the foundation for your teeth," added Apa.

Baking Soda- All of the experts agreed that baking soda is one of the strongest -- and safest -- whitening ingredients out there because it's an acid neutralizer that gently removes stains and buildup from the enamel. If this mild abrasive agent is not already mixed into your toothpaste, you can sprinkle a bit on top of your paste each day. Roth also suggested brushing with straight baking soda twice a month. "This is similar to what your dental hygienist does."

A Straw- When drinking dark beverages, like soda or grape juice, Roth suggested sipping them through a straw. "The straw allows food dyes to bypass teeth altogether."

Hydrogen Peroxide- rinsing with this antiseptic a couple of times a month can also brighten your smile, thanks to its oxidizing agents. Manymouth washes are alcohol based, but hydrogen peroxide is an antiseptic. "Mouthwash kills existing bacteria, but hydrogen peroxide prevents the growth of bacteria," said Gross. "You can gargle daily with hydrogen peroxide, but it always needs to be done in a 50/50 solution with water. Hydrogen peroxide is good for preventing infections and can also be helpful for preventing bad breath, which is often caused by bacteria."
 Mix equal parts hydrogen peroxide with water (about one tablespoon each) and swish around teeth for 60 seconds. "After a minute, spit it out, leaving the bubbling and whitening action of the peroxide to sit on teeth for another minute or two, then rinse mouth with water,"

Brush And Strip- Brushing daily with a whitening toothpaste. "Crest Weekly Clean is a good product because it contains heavy silica ingredients that work to brush stains away,".

Most over-the-counter whitening strips contain a peroxide-based whitening gel to brighten teeth, and Apa recommends Crest 2-Hour Express Whitestrips, which are made with an advanced-seal, no-slip technology that allows you to talk, drink water and go about your day .Also try rinsing your teeth with vinegar before brushing to remove tartar and prevent cavities.

Teeth Whitening:

Teeth become yellow over time
The condition can affect one's self- esteem and confidence
Causes:
Consuming tea or coffee
Excessive smoking
Neglecting oral hygiene
Aging

Natural home remedy using basil leaves and orange peels:

1. Take 6-7 crushed basil leaves
2. Add 2 tsp of dried orange peel powder
3. Mix well and make a paste
4. Apply on teeth
5. Leave it for 15 min
6. Wash off with water

Natural home remedy using baking soda:

1. Mix baking soda with water to make paste
2. Apply this paste on the teeth
3. Leave it for 3 min
4. Gargle with water
5. Do this every night at bedtime

Natural home remedy using strawberries:

1. Crush a few strawberries to make paste
2. Apply this paste on your teeth

Natural home remedy using lemon juice:

1. Remove some lemon juice
2. Apply this juice on your teeth
Tips:
Always rinse teeth after drinking tea or coffee

9 PAMPER YOUR BODY

Treating yourself to spa treatments and other luxuries are all a part of self - love. You deserve it so pamper yourself every day or at least every week. Do something for yourself that makes you happy and enjoy that moment of bliss when you're experiencing it. I speak for myself when I say that I truly enjoy doing only things that bring me happiness, bliss and joy. I also believe that every woman should do the same. Especially if you're a mother. As moms or even as wives we tend to do things to make other people happy, which is wonderful but what's not cool at all is when you lose yourself and forget the things you enjoy and stop doing what brings you happy moments. There are no excuses when it comes to spoiling yourself. If you don't feel like going to the spa you can create your own treatments at home. I will show you some self- pampering regimes in this chapter. Hey, you could even do use these techniques on people that you love and care for.

Here are a few things that I do to pamper myself at home and unwind:

I drink a lot of water throughout the day. Also I like to add slices of orange, lemon and cucumber to my water pitcher for a refreshing drink. Sometimes I add strawberries for a lightly sweet taste. At times I make my own face mask. My favorite mask to make is the olive oil, coffee and cocoa mask. Following are several face mask that I also make at home. They are all natural and are made of stuff that can be found in your kitchen. Following are a list of the face mask that I have made at home and I share with you how to make them yourselves.

Olive Oil, Coffee and Cocoa Mask

For people who have dry skin, this mask is an excellent choice. Olive oil is very similar to the oils naturally produced by your skin. So there is no need to worry about it clogging up your pores. Simply mix four tablespoons of extra virgin olive oil with two tablespoons of ground espresso and two tablespoons of cocoa powder (please be sure to choose an organic one with no whey or other dairy derivatives). Mix the ingredients to form a thick paste, and apply the mixture all over your face. Let the mask dry completely, then rinse away with warm water. The coffee and cocoa will exfoliate dead skin cells while also reducing puffiness, leaving your complexion looking bright and clean.

Orange Juice, Olive Oil and Avocado

 This is like my second favorite mask, you guys. Avocados are rich in an assortment of essential vitamins and nutrients, including vitamin K and vitamin E. Combined with the vitamin C naturally found in oranges and the hydrating properties of olive oil, this is a great mask for combination skin. Simply mash a ripe avocado and mix with a teaspoon of fresh squeezed orange juice from an orange and a teaspoon of extra virgin olive oil. Spread the mixture over your face and allow it to set in for 20 minutes before rinsing it off with warm water.

Strawberries and Rice Milk

Salicylic acid is one of the most popular ingredients in over-the-counter face washes, and strawberries are a natural source of it. Personally I like to eat strawberries. It's totally my favorite fruit to consume. If you have acne-prone skin, this is one of the best masks you can make at home. Simply mash six strawberries and add 1/2 tablespoon of organic rice milk to make a paste. Apply it to your skin and allow it to set for 15 minutes before rinsing it away with warm water. The strawberries will help clear up acne and blemishes while the rice milk will help hydrate dull, dry skin.

Oatmeal and Soy Yogurt

This is more like a vegan mask is suitable for all skin types and takes only a few seconds to prepare. Simply combine a tablespoon of organic oatmeal with a tablespoon of soy yogurt and mix the two ingredients together to make a paste. Apply the paste to your face and allow it to set for 10 minutes, then rinse away with warm water. The oats will help exfoliate your pores while also absorbing excess oil while the soy yogurt helps hydrate your skin.

After I've got my facial mask on, I like to listen to some relaxing to music. I love classical music, from Beethoven to Mozart. Hey, whatever type of music that you find relaxing is fine. As long as you feel truly relaxed. The idea is to feel as you would at the spa, at home. Then I fill the bath tub with warm coconut milk and light scented candles. Once I hop in that tub, I feel like I'm in a different world, one of which I do not want to ever leave. If you're not into bathing in coconut milk you can prepare a special bath. Here's another bath that I've prepared and tried, I actually enjoyed it.

Stress Free Relieving Bath

Draw a hot bath with a few bath salts of your choice . The natural mineral blend has lavender, chamomile, St. John's Worth, valerian and hops to relax and detox your body. It also has oils (sunflower and olive), but not too much so I would recommend it for normal, combination or oily skin. Then use a body wash and a pouf or loofah to scrub away dead skin. Rub it in a circular motion, for a more effective result. There are a ton of good, natural body washes out there. You can use a gel to scrub while you're sitting in the bath tub and it will add more bubbles to your bath. Please fun, if you ask me. When I am in the bath I like to meditate, it's so much more serene and relaxing. Once you're done, dry your body lightly while still leaving some moisture on your skin. Before your skin is completely dry, rub on some body oil. My favorite is chamomile or cherry oil. Lather it on everywhere it won't clog pores. Do not put it on your face. However I think it would be fine to apply the oil to dry facial skin. You can also use regular body lotion if you prefer it, but the body oil is nice for a deep moisture. Whichever kind you use, putting it on when your skin is slightly damp means you'll absorb more moisture. Always use a deep moisturizer on your face. Even if you have oily skin, you need moisture. I like to use a deep moisturizer every now and then. I just put natural cocoa butter, shea butter or avocado on my face. It's pretty heavy, so I would only use this at night before bed time. I see it as a special treat for my skin. Since I live in a cold, windy climate, I use this every day. Once I am in my night gown and I've applied my moisturizer, I then make myself one of many healthy drinks. My favorite is a pomegranate martini. Anyway, following I will share with you a few of my healthy tasty drinks and how to make them.

Pomegranate Martini

You'll need:
1 bottle of Ketel One Citroen Flavored Vodka
pomegranate liqueur
fresh lemon sour
pomegranate juice
1 small piece of orange peel

How to Mix
Glass: Martini Glass
Shake with ice in a cocktail shaker.
Serve straight up in a martini glass.
Garnish with an orange twist.
Fresh Lemon Sour: 4 oz fresh lemon juice.
2 oz simple syrup.
5 oz water.
Combine all ingredients and stir well
Then you're ready to begin sipping.

Blueberry-Lime Margarita

You'll need:
2 cups ice
1 cup frozen blueberries
1 cup blueberry nectar
1/4 cup seltzer
2 tablespoons frozen limeade
1 tablespoon lime juice
3 ounces tequila, optional
1 lime wedge
Coarse salt

How to Mix
Combine ice, blueberries, blueberry nectar, seltzer, limeade, lime juice and tequila, if using, in a blender and blend until smooth. Rub rim of 2 glasses with lime wedge and dip in salt. Divide the margarita between the prepared glasses and serve.

Island Limeade

You'll need:
3 cups boiling water
1/3-1/2 cup sugar
1 1/4 cups freshly squeezed lime juice
6 ounces dark rum

How to mix
Combine boiling water and sugar to taste. Stir until the sugar dissolves; chill. Add the lime juice to make limeade. Fill 4 tall glasses with ice and divide the rum among the glasses. Top with the limeade. Non-alcoholic variation: Omit the rum.

The following is a drink that is made with ginger in. Peeled ginger keeps very well for months in the fridge, if you submerge it in a high-quality, high proof alcohol. Just peel the ginger and break it into manageable pieces and then pour vodka or vermouth or even sherry (though vodka is best). If you're planning on using it to cook with, the alcohol will just cook right off when you do. Bonus: You'll have ginger-infused vodka to make a new, fancy martini with.

Here are some soothing foot bath that you can prepare at home:

Mustard-Ginger Detoxifying and De-stressing Foot Soak

A long-famed traditional home remedy for aches, colds, chills, and general fatigue and sickness, mustard foot baths are the bomb for the days or nights where you just don't feel up to it.

Add a little fresh ground ginger in with it, and you've got yourself a foot bath that will help warm you, relax the muscles in your feet, and detoxify your system straight through the soles.

You don't need a fancy foot bath like I have. Just fill your bathtub (or another large foot-sized basin) up with very warm water and add your ingredients.

Remember, hot water "deactivates" mustard, making it milder and not as potent. So it's best to do your mustard-ginger foot baths in warm water, not piping hot.

Mustard-Ginger Foot Bath Recipe

1-1/2tsp mustard powder (or freshly powdered mustard seeds)
2 tsp finely grated peeled fresh ginger
Combine the two in a basin that fits your feet (or your bathtub) with enough hot water to cover the tops of your feet. Stir around and then submerge your feet. Let your feet soak for 15-20 minutes, swishing the water around occasionally (and adding more warm water, if your foot bath becomes too cold). Rinse with warm water and pat dry.

Here are some baths and massage oils that you can prepare:

Romantic, Warming Ginger-Rose Massage Oil

Don't wait until Valentine's Day guys! And if you start a batch of this now, you should be good to go by the big day. I can't think of a better gift for you and your significant other that you can both enjoy (regardless of who's doing the massaging).
The only thing you should note with this: If you're making it the old-fashioned way, by infusing the oil over time, you might want to use a few drops of rosemary essential oil in the mixture, just to keep it well preserved. Ginger isn't a very watery ingredient, but fresh ginger does contain moisture, so be careful that it doesn't go rancid or start to mold a little.

I've been infusing mine for three days, and it looks great. Ginger's also highly antibacterial and antifungal, so you should be okay. When in doubt, add extra preservatives (or use the less-intense dried ginger).
Alternatively, you could infuse the oil over low heat with the ginger and rosebuds, and then use it immediately.

Rose Ginger Romantic Massage Oil

1 inch peeled, completely clean piece of ginger root, cut into thin slices
10-12 small dried rosebuds
1 cup of coconut oil (sweet almond, olive, jojoba, hazelnut, etc.)
In a small glass container, combine all ingredients and shake to combine, knocking on the side of the glass until all the ginger falls to the bottom. Either let this concoction sit for 5-7 days, shaking daily, or heat over very low heat for 30 minutes to an hour. Use as a warming, romantic massage oil. But keep out of delicate places, because ginger is pretty intense.
A little note, ginger is also an exceptional muscle ache reliever. So you don't just have to use this for sexy times. Use it whenever you feel tired or have a sore muscle.

Cozy Ginger-Cinnamon Bath Salts

For this last idea, you can use either coarsely ground sea salt, like I did, or up the ante for relieving muscle aches by using Epsom salts.
Both ginger and cinnamon encourage good circulation, which in turn helps relieve some of the aches and pains you may feel after a long day. But even better, their scents are so homey and relaxing, so you'll drift away into relaxation before you know it.

Warming Cinnamon-Ginger Bath Salts

1/4 cup of coarsely ground sea salt or Epsom salts
3 tsp peeled, finely ground or grated ginger
1/2 tsp ground cinnamon
5 drops sweet orange essential oil (optional, for even more relaxation)
Combine all ingredients in a small container and stir well. Add to your hot bath, and swish around a bit before getting in. Soak for 15-20 minutes. Use immediately.

Another soothing bath is to add 2 or 3 cups of apple cider vinegar to your bath water and soak to relieve tired achy muscles and this will help eliminate yeast infections. Apple cider vinegar will help balance your body's pH levels.

10 NATURAL BREAST ENHANCEMENT

A breast implant is a prosthesis used to correct the size, form, and texture of a woman's breast; in plastic surgery, breast implants are applied for post–mastectomy breast reconstruction; for correcting congenital defects and deformities of the chest wall; for aesthetic breast augmentation; and for creating breasts in the male to female transsexual patient. There are three general types of breast implant devices, defined by their filler material: saline solution, silicone gel, and composite filler. The saline implant has an elastomer silicone shell filled with sterile saline solution; the silicone implant has an elastomer silicone shell filled with viscous silicone gel; and the alternative composition implants featured miscellaneous fillers, such as soy oil, polypropylene string, et cetera. In surgical practice, for the reconstruction of a breast, the tissue expander device is a temporary breast prosthesis used to form and establish an implant pocket for emplacing the permanent breast implant.

In the 19th century
Since the late nineteenth century, breast implants have been used to surgically augment the size (volume), modify the shape (contour), and enhance the feel (tact) of a woman's breasts. In 1895, surgeon Vincenz Czerny effected the earliest breast implant emplacement when he used the patient's autologous adipose tissue, harvested from a benign lumbar lipoma, to repair the asymmetry of the breast from which he had removed a tumor. In 1889, surgeon Robert Gersuny experimented with paraffin injections, with disastrous results. From the first half of the twentieth century, physicians used other substances as breast implant fillers ivory, glass balls, ground rubber, ox cartilage, Terylene wool, gutta percha, Dicora, polyethylene chips, Ivalon (polyvinyl alcohol formaldehyde polymer sponge), a polyethylene sac with Ivalon, polyether foam sponge (Etheron), polyethylene tape (Polystan) strips wound into a ball, polyester (polyurethane foam sponge) Silastic rubber, and teflon silicone prostheses.

In The 20th century

In the mid-twentieth century, Morton I. Berson, in 1945, and Jacques Maliniac, in 1950, each performed flap-based breast augmentations by rotating the patient's chest wall tissue into the breast to increase its volume. Furthermore, throughout the 1950s and the 1960s, plastic surgeons used synthetic fillers including silicone injections received by some 50,000 women, from which developed silicone granulomas and breast hardening that required treatment by mastectomy. In 1961, the American plastic surgeons Thomas Cronin and Frank Gerow, and the Dow Corning Corporation, developed the first silicone breast prosthesis, filled with silicone gel; in due course, the first augmentation mamoplasty was performed in 1962 using the Cronin Gerow Implant, prosthesis model 1963. In 1964, the French company Laboratories Arion developed and manufactured the saline breast implant, filled with saline solution, and then introduced for use as a medical device in 1964. There are many different types of breast augmentation. They are the saline implant filled with sterile saline solution. The silicone implant filled with viscous silicone gel. Then you have the alternative-composition implant with miscellaneous fillers (e.g. soy oil, polypropylene string, etc.) that are no longer manufactured.

Saline Implants

A saline breast implant is comprised of a silicone elastomer shell or bag filled with a sterile saline solution.

Silicone Implants

A breast implant is a prosthesis used to correct the size, form, and texture of a woman's breast; in plastic surgery, breast implants are applied for post–mastectomy breast reconstruction; for correcting congenital defects and deformities of the chest wall; for aesthetic breast augmentation

What's the difference between saline and silicone breast implants?
Saline and silicone breast implants both have an outer silicone shell. The implants differ in material and consistency, however.

Saline breast implants

Saline implants are filled with sterile salt water. They're inserted empty, and then filled once they're in place.
Saline breast implants are available to women 18 and older for breast augmentation and to women of any age for breast reconstruction.

Silicone breast implants

Silicone implants are pre-filled with silicone gel, a thick, sticky fluid that closely mimics the feel of human fat. Most women feel that silicone breast implants look and feel more like natural breast tissue.
Silicone breast implants are available to women 22 and older for breast augmentation and to women of any age for breast reconstruction.

What are the risks of breast implants?

Saline and silicone breast implants pose similar risks, including:

Scar tissue that distorts the shape of the breast implant (capsular contracture)
Breast pain
Infection
Changes in nipple and breast sensation, usually temporary
Implant leakage or rupture
Correcting any of these complications might require additional surgery, either to remove or replace the implants.

What happens if an implant ruptures?

If an implant ruptures, the approach might vary depending on whether the implant is saline or silicone.

Ruptured saline implant

If a saline breast implant ruptures, the implant will deflate causing the affected breast to change in size and shape.
The leaking saline solution will be absorbed by your body without posing any health risks, but you'll probably need surgery to remove the silicone shell. If you wish, a new implant can likely be inserted at the same time.

Ruptured silicone implant

If a silicone breast implant ruptures, you might not notice right away or ever because any free silicone tends to remain trapped in the fibrous tissue (capsule) that forms around the implant. This is known as a silent rupture. Leaking silicone gel isn't thought to cause systemic or long-term health problems such as breast cancer, reproductive problems or connective tissue disease, such as rheumatoid arthritis. Still, a ruptured silicone breast implant might eventually cause breast pain or changes in the contour or shape of the breast.
If this happens, your doctor will likely recommend surgical removal. If you wish, a new implant can usually be inserted at the same time.
If an MRI scan detects an implant rupture but you don't have any signs or symptoms, it might be up to you and your doctor to weigh the risks and benefits of keeping the implant in place or having it removed.

Breast Enlargement:

Estrogen facilitates breast growth during puberty
Small breast size can affect a woman's self esteem
Nutrition and genetics also play an important role in determining the size of breasts.

Natural home remedy using fenugreek powder:

1. Fenugreek has properties which helps grow breast size and also makes them firm
2. Take ¼ bowl of fenugreek powder
3. Add a little water
4. Mix well to make a paste
5. Apply this on the breasts
6. Massage gently
7. Leave for 15-20 minutes
8. Wash off with water

Natural home remedy using cod liver oil and fennel seeds:

1. Fennel seeds have flavonoids which facilitate growth of breast tissue
2. Heat cod liver oil in a pan
3. Add 2 tsp of fennel seeds
4. Allow fennel seeds to turn red
5. Strain the oil
6. Apply this oil on the breasts
7. Massage gently
8. Wash off after 30 min
9. Do this every day

11 INFALLIBLE DIETING

First, I would like to make it very clear to you that I am not a nutritionist, health care professional and I'm not a specialist either. Please consult with your doctor before stating any dieting. With that said, you may try the diets in this chapter at your own risk. There are so many diets out there. I should know since I am always on a diet. It's really nerve racking at times. I honestly could tell you how it is that my body gains weight because I am really not a fast food eater at all but perhaps processed food, even in small amounts might have and incredible effect on my body in a negative way. The funny thing is every year I go on this very unhealthy diet (fast), that actually works. Then I lose a ton of weight and like six or seven months later, I'm back to square one all over again. So as I'm writing this book now, I'm on a eighty day liquid fast which I will have to extend to one hundred and twenty days, rather than the eighty days because this time I want to actually maintain the results this time. If it means that I could never eat rice, bread or any form of carbohydrate, then I'm willing to make the sacrifice. There are so many diets that work but the problem is maintaining the healthy weight once we've achieved it. I would like to share with you some weight loss solutions that are not as drastic like the unhealthy fast that I am currently one.

Home Remedies to lose weight

Fennel - Has been used since ancient times to reduce appetite and was traditionally used to prevent 'growling stomachs' during church services!.

Peppermint - Is an herb of the mint family and has been used for hundreds of years to promote healthy digestion. Relax the muscles of the digestive tract and stimulates the natural flow of digestive juices and bile, thereby assisting the body to digest and process food efficiently. Peppermint has also been shown to facilitate healthy digestion by calming the stomach.

Dandelion - Is particularly nutritious. It contains substantial levels of vitamins A, C, D, and B complex and iron, magnesium, zinc, potassium, manganese, copper, choline, calcium, boron and silicon. The bitter principle of dandelion stimulates digestion, including the secretion of salivary and gastric juices.

Licorice - Originates in the Mediterranean and the Middle East and has many uses, including being a general tonic for the digestive system. A recent human study found that a preparation of licorice may reduce body fat. Fifteen people of normal weight consumed licorice for 2 months (3.5 g per day). The mass of body fat was measured before and after treatment. Licorice reduced the mass of body fat and suppressed the hormone aldosterone. Another study found that a topical preparation of glycyrrhetinic acid (a component of licorice) could reduce the thickness of fat in the thigh in humans.

Fruits and vegetables that burn fat

Apples

An apple a day helps keep fat away. apples contain lots of vitamin c, which dilutes fat and makes it easier to flush from the body. Apples also have pectin, a complex carbohydrate that limits the amount of fat absorbed into cells. Pectin even aids with water absorption, again helping flush fat.

Asparagus

The alkaline chemical asparagine, found in asparagus, helps break down fat and stimulates the kidneys, improving the overall circulatory process. Asparagus also destroys the oxalic acid that glues fat to cells, allowing the fat to be removed from the system before it has a chance to be stored in the body.

Broccoli

A true super food, broccoli contains scores of vitamins and nutrients, including high levels of vitamin c, vitamin a, folic acid and calcium. Broccoli's fiber content forces the body to expend more energy during digestion, making it a highly effective fat-burner. Add in its disease-fighting antioxidants, and broccoli deserves a spot on every dinner plate.

Brussels Sprouts

Brussels sprouts are high in fat-burning components like vitamin c and fiber, and also have a combination of minerals that stimulate the glands into releasing hormones that cleanse cells of fat. The leafy green vegetables also stimulate the kidneys, helping more fat to be flushed from the body.

Carrots

Carrots get their distinctive orange coloring from carotene, a form of vitamin a. Carotene prompts a fat-flushing reaction within the body. Once inside the intestines, carotene also transforms into vitamin a, helping raise the body's metabolism and burn more calories.

Oranges

Thanks to their high vitamin c content, oranges provide excellent fat-burning potential. oranges also contain pulp and fiber, which require the body to spend more energy on digestion. As a result, more calories get burned, resulting in fat reduction. other citrus fruits, such as limes and lemons, deliver the same fat-burning benefits.

Peppers

Peppers, and in particular chili peppers, contain capsaicin, the chemical compound that gives them their heat. once ingested, capsaicin forces the body to produce more stress hormones, leading to an increase in metabolic rate and more expended calories. Mixing some cayenne pepper into fatty foods can help negate the caloric intake.

Grapefruit

Eating grapefruit can help you burn belly fat. this citrus fruit is rich in vitamin c, a vitamin that can strengthen your immune system, increase your metabolism and dilute fats. Other helpful fruits rich in vitamin c are limes, lemons, tangerines and oranges.

Low-fat dairy

Adding calcium-rich, low-fat dairy foods into your daily diet can help you burn belly fat. Dairy foods such as low-fat milk, skim milk, low-fat cheese and plain reduced-fat yogurt can boost weight loss by breaking down accumulated fat in your fat cells. A calcium deficiency can trigger the release of calcitriol which is a hormone that stores fat in your body.

Chilies and cayenne peppers

Iif you want to burn belly fat, add spicy chilies or cayenne peppers to your daily diet. these spicy vegetables contain capsaicin, a chemical compound that increases your metabolism, encourages weight loss and increases your energy level. According to fat free kitchen, foods rich in capsaicin can continue to burn calories up to 20 minutes after eating them.

Protein-based foods

Eating protein-based foods can boost your metabolism and help you shed excess belly fat. It takes more energy to digest protein-based foods, such as turkey, fish, chicken, beans, eggs, soy and tofu, than it does to digest fats and carbohydrates, meaning you burn more calories digesting these foods.

Lentils

If you want to flatten your belly, add lentils into your daily diet. According to fat free kitchen, lentils are rich in protein and soluble fiber, nutrients that stimulate your metabolism, stabilize your blood sugar levels and increase your body's fat-burning abilities.

Peanuts

If you want to burn unwanted belly fat, try snacking on peanuts. Peanuts are loaded with fiber, protein and healthy unsaturated fat. They prevent weight gain, stabilize blood sugar levels and delay the feeling of hunger.

Oatmeal

Oatmeal contains soluble fiber that helps flush digestive acids out of your system, allowing you to feel satiated for a longer amount of time. Oatmeal also helps lower your blood cholesterol levels and decrease your risk of developing colon cancer or heart disease.

Natural Appetite Suppressants

Almonds- Just a handful of almonds is a rich source of antioxidants, vitamin e, and magnesium. Almonds have also been shown to increase feelings of fullness in people and help with weight management, according to a study presented at the 2006 obesity society annual scientific meeting. So what are you waiting for? Munch on almonds for your next healthy snack!

Coffee- While drinking more than one to two cups of Joe a day can leave you feeling jittery and nervous, a moderate amount of coffee can help boost metabolism and suppress your appetite. Coffee's secret? Caffeine, along with antioxidants from the coffee beans. Just don't cancel out those good effects with too much sugar or cream!

Ginger- For centuries, many cultures have used ginger root for its amazing digestive powers. Whether it's in a smoothie or in an Indian dish (sorry, ginger ale doesn't count!), ginger works as a stimulant that energizes the body and improves digestion, thereby making you less hungry.

Avocado- Full of fiber and heart-healthy monounsaturated fat, avocados suppress appetite when eaten in moderation. In fact, the fats in these little guys send signals to your brain that tell your stomach that it's full!

Cayenne Pepper- Get spicy! According to recent research published in the journal physiology & behavior, just half a teaspoon of cayenne pepper can boost metabolism and cause the body to burn an extra 10 calories on its own. Not to mention that for those who don't regularly eat spicy meals, adding cayenne pepper cuts an average of 60 calories from their next meal. Do that at two meals a day for a month and you'll lose 4 pounds without even trying!

Apples- Apples of all varieties and types help suppress hunger for a number of reasons. First, apples are filled with soluble fiber and pectin, which help you feel full. Apples also regulate your glucose and boost your energy level. Finally, apples require lots of chewing time, which helps slow you down and gives your body more time to realize that you're no longer hungry. Plus, they just taste good!

Eggs- Studies have shown that eating an egg or two for breakfast can help dieters feel more full over 24 hours than if they eat a bagel with the same amount of calories. In the same study, those who ate eggs ingested an average of 330 fewer calories over the course of a day than the bagel-eaters.

Food for thought?

Water- Could taming your appetite be as easy as drinking an extra glass or two of water? Science says yes! In August of 2010 a study showed that people who drank two glasses of water before a meal ate between 75 and 90 fewer calories at the meal than those who didn't drink water. Love that H2O!

Sweet Potatoes- According to food scientists, potatoes contain a special type of starch that resists digestive enzymes, making them stay in your stomach longer and therefore keep you full. plus, they're full of vitamin a and vitamin c!

Umeboshi Plums- Have a sweet craving you just can't shake? Sometimes the best thing to do is to shock it with something sour. Umeboshi Plums are basically pickled plums and can be fantastic for squashing sugar cravings. Find them at your local specialty store or asian grocer.

Vegetable Soup- A hot, broth-based vegetable soup can fill you up in a hurry and take the edge off of your hunger with minimal calories. Try having a cup before your next meal or simply have a big bowl as your main course!

Dark Chocolate- Love chocolate but have no self- control with it? Try slowly savoring a piece or two of dark chocolate with at least 70 percent cocoa the next time you crave it. just a little dark chocolate helps to lower your cravings because the bitter taste signals the body to decrease your appetite. Not to mention that the steric acid in dark chocolate helps slow digestion to help you feel fuller longer. If dark chocolate is too bitter for you, try having a piece with a cup of black coffee it'll bring out the sweetness!

Tofu- A rich plant-based protein source, tofu isn't just for vegetarians! Tofu is high in an Iso-flavone called Genistein, which has been shown to suppress appetite and lower food intake. For an easy way to introduce tofu in your diet, try adding it to your next healthy stir-fry.

Wasabi- Ever notice how when you eat sushi it doesn't seem to take as much food to fill you up? Well, part of that is because of the healthy fish in sushi, but the other part is due to that spicy green stuff: wasabi! The spiciness in wasabi suppresses appetite and is a natural anti-inflammatory.

Green Tea- If you're not a coffee drinker and get sick of water easily, try sipping on a cup of hot green tea. Green tea can help you to stop mindlessly snacking, and nutritionists say that the catechins in green tea help to inhibit the movement of glucose into fat cells, which slows the rise of blood sugar and prevents high insulin and subsequent fat storage and when your blood sugar is more stable so is your hunger!

Oatmeal- Did this one surprise you? While high in carbs, the type of carbs in oatmeal are slow-digesting and keep you feeling full for hours after breakfast. Why? Because they suppress the hunger hormone ghrelin. In fact, oatmeal is pretty low on the glycemic index, just be sure to make steel cut oats to get the most benefit!

Vegetable Juice- You probably think that vegetable juice is just a way to get more veggies in your diet, right? That's true, but veggie juice has also been shown to fill you up. In fact, when people drank vegetable juice before a meal, they ended up eating 135 fewer calories. Now that's some appetite suppression! Just be sure to drink the low-sodium varieties, which are less likely to make you bloat.

Green Leafy Vegetables- If you're really looking for a highly nutritious food that will fill you up for hours, you can't beat green leafy vegetables. From kale to spinach to Swiss chard, these fibrous greens (eaten raw or gently sautéed with a little olive oil) are delicious and definitely keep hunger at bay.

Salmon- When you eat fish like salmon that are high in omega-3 fatty acids, your body increases the amount of the hormone leptin in your system. Leptin is known for suppressing hunger. Don't like salmon? Try tuna and herring, which are also high in omega-3s!

Cinnamon- Next time you have cereal, oatmeal, fruit, or even coffee, sprinkle some cinnamon on it. Cinnamon, like other ground spices such as cloves and ginger, helps lower your blood sugar levels, which you guessed, it helps to control your appetite!

Skim Milk- If PMS cravings have your hunger all out of whack during that time of the month, try drinking skim milk. Studies show that women who have at least one serving of dairy a day about two weeks before menstruation significantly decrease their cravings for unhealthy junk foods and processed carbs.

Hot Sauce- When it comes to hot sauce and appetite suppression, the hotter you can go the better. So get some Tabasco and sprinkle some heat on your burrito, scrambled eggs, or even soup! The spiciness keeps you from overeating and helps you to stay full longer.

Flax Seeds- With a nutritional mix of soluble fiber and essential fatty acids, flax seeds are the perfect addition to your yogurt, smoothie, or salad. In fact, ground or whole, flax seeds help you to stay satiated and fueled!

Salad- If you want to keep the hunger monster from rearing its food-devouring head, eat a small salad before you sit down for a meal. Just a cup or two of veggies is all it takes to signal to your brain that you're getting calories and nutrition. Since it takes about 20 minutes for your stomach to signal to your brain that you're full, starting with a small salad before your meal, is a perfect way to get a head-start on that hunger signal.

Whey Protein- Protein is known for suppressing appetite, but it seems that whey protein is especially good at it. New research shows that after people have a liquid meal with whey protein they consume significantly fewer calories at their next meal than those who had a liquid meal with casein protein. Stock up on whey protein at your local natural foods store to reap this benefit!

Weight Loss:
Being overweight is harmful to one's self esteem.
It is also a health concern since it leads to many serious ailments including:
  Diabetes
  High blood pressure

Causes:
Some people overeat when they are:
  Depressed
  Bored
  Angry
  In a relaxed environment
  Incorrect lifestyle
  Improper diet
  Lack of exercise
  Hypothyroidism

Natural home remedy using black pepper powder, lemon juice and honey:

1. Take 1 glass lukewarm water
2. Add 1 tsp black pepper powder
3. Add 4 tbsp lemon juice
4. Add 1 tsp honey
5. Mix well
6. Drink every day

Natural home remedy using lemon juice and honey:

1. Take 1 glass hot water
2. Add 4 tbsp lemon juice
3. Add 1 tbsp honey
4. Drink every morning on empty stomach
Tips:
Exercise regularly
Cabbage is very effective in burning body fat. Consume 1 bowl of cabbage every day.

The 3 Day Diet

The 3 Day Diet, also referred to as the Cardiac Diet, is meant for rapid weight loss. It is often used in hospitals for cardiac patients who need to lose large amounts of weight before having heart surgery.

Proponents of this diet claim that you can drop 10 pounds in three days and that you can manage to lose 40 pounds in one month.

Being extremely low in calories, it is unhealthy to follow this diet for more than 3 days. After the 3 day period, you should return to your normal food intake for about four to five days. Only then you can repeat this diet again.

This diet consists of eating moderate portions of tuna, lean meat, grapefruit, toast, eggs and vegetables. Portions must be eaten exactly as specified in the diet plan. Only salt, pepper, and ketchup can be used to season foods and no sugar is allowed. Dieters are encouraged to drink 8 glasses of water a day.

The 3 Day Diet Meal Plan:

Day 1

Breakfast:
Black coffee or tea, with 1-2 packets Sweet & Low or Equal
½ grapefruit or juice
1 piece toast with 1 tablespoon peanut butter

Lunch:
½ cup tuna
1 piece toast
Black coffee or tea, with 1-2 packets Sweet & Low or Equal

Dinner:
3 ounces any lean meat or chicken
1 cup green beans
1 cup carrots
1 apple
1 cup regular vanilla ice cream

Day 2

Breakfast:
Black coffee or tea, with 1-2 packets Sweet & Low or Equal
1 egg
½ banana
1 piece toast

Lunch:
1 cup cottage cheese or tuna
8 regular saltine crackers or 1 piece toast

Dinner:
2 beef franks
1 cup broccoli or cabbage
½ cup carrots
½ banana
½ cup regular vanilla ice cream

Day 3

Breakfast:
Black coffee or tea, with 1-2 packets Sweet & Low or Equal
5 regular saltine crackers
1 ounce cheddar cheese
1 apple

Lunch:
Black coffee or tea, with 1-2 packets Sweet & low or equal
1 boiled egg
1 piece toast

Dinner:
1 cup tuna
1 cup carrots
1 cup cauliflower
1 cup melon
½ cup regular vanilla ice cream

Garlic Process

Here is a diet regime that I have done several times in the past and it has worked each time and given me excellent results. I call it the "garlic process". Ok, so you would pick three consecutive days. For example: start on a Wednesday morning by taking to cloves of garlic and cutting those two cloves of garlic into little pieces. Next you'll fill a glass 3/4 of lukewarm water or room temperature water and then you will place the chopped garlic pieces into the glass. Leave the glass covered all day and on that very same night, you'll strain the garlic water and drink the water. Afterwards you'll cut another two cloves of garlic and full a glass with water again and place the chopped little garlic pieces into the glass. Cover the glass and leave it overnight. When you wake up on the Thursday morning you're going to strain the garlic water and drink the water without the garlic. Then you'll get another two cloves of garlic and cut them into little pieces and place it in a glass with water, cover it and leave it until Friday morning. On Friday morning, strain the garlic water and drink it. You may repeat the same process on the following week or as many weeks as you need ,until you've achieved your desired weight.
Note: To get rid of garlic breath, just drink some milk or gargle with milk. This garlic process has been one of the most effective diets that I have gone on and it has worked. By the way, I forgot to mention that you could still eat a healthy diet and lose weight while doing the garlic process.

A Couple More Tips:

WHAT IS WAIST TRAINING ?

Waist training is a gradual process of waist reduction using a corset. Also known as waist cinching, this practice came to prominence during the Victorian times. I love it because it helps to give me an "hour glass figure." Waist training requires dedication and devotion, it is not something that will just happen by occasionally wearing your corset and it will take time, it will also need maintenance. I have been asked if a corset will permanently reduce your waist by however many inches, the corset is an inanimate object, it won't do anything unless you use it to do what you want it to do. The key factor here is your discipline and dedication.

The more you wear a corset that pulls in your waist, the more effect it will have. Waist reduction and reshaping requires discipline. The best results are achieved with combining these key factors waist cinching using your corset to pull in your waist as much as possible. Be sure to follow a healthy diet, drink lots of water and regular exercise.

Drink Water throughout out the day

When your skin becomes dehydrated it loses It's firm appearance. The elasticity of the skin slackens therefore hydrating the skin is key. Aim to drink more than eight glasses of water each day.

Food as Lifting Therapy

Eat food that encourages the skin to repair itself and help tone. Eat food such as protein found in chicken, fish, nuts, low fat cottage cheese and yogurt.

Carotenoid pigments found in food are believed to contribute to a healthy skin glow. Include foods in your diet such as carrots, yams, spinach, peaches, pumpkin, apricots, watermelons, tomatoes, pink grapefruit and apricots.

Eat a rainbow of fruit because fruit contain antioxidants called flavonoids and carotenoids, these will remove the free radicals from your skin that cause the skin to age prematurely.

Exercise

I am not the greatest fan of exercise but I will say that I do enjoy doing lots of cardio, pilates and yoga. What helps me to enjoy cardio and pilates is music. I enjoy working out to samba and modern day soca music. It really gets me going. You should try it out. When you begin to workout, you'll feel some pain for about the first two weeks but once you've overcome that part and you work out on a regular basis, let's like at least 4-5 days a week. You'll definitely tone up and lose lots of fat. To increase the fat burn, I drink 3-4 tablespoons of organic apple cider vinegar before I work out. It melts fat so quickly and gives me so much energy. That energy also helps me to enjoy each workout and it also helps to keep me motivated as well. Eventually exercise will become a normal part of your daily routine. So no excuses you guys. There is no such thing as, " I don't have the time". Make time! Even if it's thirty minutes a day, 6-7 times a week. Just do it!

Toning Exercise

Cardio exercise alone won't tone the muscles you need to add some weight resistant exercises to help bulk the muscles and fill out the loose skin. Toned muscles help to create the appearance of tight lifted youthful skin.

Healthy drinks

This is a quick on the run smoothie recipe that will take minutes to make, will leave the kitchen with little mess and is delicious.

This smoothie is made of the king of all fruits mango, using natural yogurt and crushed ice which is perfect for warmer weather days.

How to make (for 2 small glasses)

1 medium mango

1 cup of yogurt

handful of crushed ice

Cut the mango by separating the flesh from the mango and removing the pit.

Cut the mango into cubes.

Place mango and yogurt into blender and blend until smooth.

Add the crushed ice and enjoy

Some of the health and skin benefits of eating Probiotic Mango Smoothie:

Mango benefits

Rich source of iron

High amounts of anti-ageing antioxidants and helps to fight against cancers and heart disease

Boosts memory

Helps clear clogged pores so useful for acne and combination skin types

A good source of potassium which is important for cell and body fluids, helping to cure a hangover

The Bio-active elements of mango such as Esters, Terpenes and Aldehydes aids digestion

Helps regulate the sex hormones and boosts sex drive

Yogurt Benefits

Soothes the stomach, reduces bloating and encourages healthy bacteria growth in colon.

A rich source of calcium which helps to decrease the risk of colon cancer full of protein and vitamin d helping to strengthen bones, fight depression and boost immunity.

All of these healthy benefits in one delicious drink.

Pumpkin

Pumpkin and its seeds is one of the best beauty super foods. The alpha and beta-carotene found in pumpkins are potent antioxidants keeping your skin looking firm and youthful. they are packed full of vitamins and zinc helping to boost immunity, protect your cell membranes, maintain collagen, and promote skin renewal; making it one of the best skin treatments inside and out!

Here are some of my favorite beauty pumpkin recipes:

Pumpkin Brew

serves: 4
prep: 10 mins | cook: 40 mins

Ingredients

1 teaspoon olive oil
1 medium sized pumpkin cut and cubed (keep the seeds for roasting)
1 onion
1 small potato
1 celery
1 carrot
2 pints of water with veg stock
¼ teaspoon of ground ginger
1 teaspoon of thyme
¼ cup parmesan cheese
salt and pepper to taste

Instructions

In a large saucepan, sauté onion in olive oil until tender. add ginger and thyme and cook for 30 seconds. add pumpkin cubes, potato, carrot, water and continue to heat until thickened; whilst heating continue to the roasted pumpkin seeds recipe.

Puree in a food processor and return to saucepan.

Remove from heat and sprinkle with the roasted pumpkin seeds and parmesan cheese.

Season with salt and pepper.

Roasted Pumpkin Seeds

serves: 4
prep: 5 mins | cook: 15 mins

Ingredients

150g (5 oz) pumpkin seeds
1 tablespoon olive oil
1/2 teaspoon salt
instructions
1. Preheat the oven to 140 c / gas mark 1. line a baking tray with baking parchment or foil.
2. Prepare pumpkin seeds: rinse with water, and remove any strings and bits of squash. pat dry, and place in a small bowl.
2. Stir the olive oil and salt into the seeds until evenly coated. spread out in an even layer on the prepared baking tray.
3. Bake for 15 minutes, or until seeds start to pop. remove from oven and cool on the baking tray before serving.

ABOUT THE AUTHOR

My name is Karen Vincent. I am an
author, business woman and much more. I am in my twenties. Also I
grew up in South America and first visited the United States at the age of
five. I eventually came to the states to live at the age of fourteen. For
someone
so young, I have lived a very interesting life and have endured quite a lot.
I have written a book about my life which will soon be published.
In the book which I wrote about my life, I share many different
experiences some good and some less wonderful ones. I felt the need to
write that book so that young ladies especially my daughter can learn
from my mistakes, life experiences. Also I wrote the book in hopes of
being able to reach young ladies all over the world to show them that
they too can achieve anything they want if they just work hard towards it.
There is a lot to me and my persona. Too much to write in this book
but as time goes by and with every book that I write I hope to be able to
reach more and more people.
As far as the type of personality I have, I am very
outgoing, selfless, caring, ambitious, kind ,loving and intelligent young
lady. I also have much knowledge to share with the world.
I really hate writing about myself but I feel the need to let you know
more about me. Also it is my obligation as the author of a book which
you purchased to give you a better sense of who I am and to be honest
with you. I hope to build a relationship with my readers as time goes by.
At times I can be really forward but trust me it comes from a good
place and with very good intentions.

Writing is one of my callings in this life. It is one
of the things that I was sent on this earth to do and I look forward to
doing it well.
Please, if you have any constructive criticism for me, I will accept it.
Just as well I would love to accept any compliments which you might
have for me. I have added my contact information where I can be
reached.
So please feel free to contact me either way. I appreciate your
comments. It is important for me as an author to be able to connect with
my readers and give you quality content in my books. My readers mean
the world to me and please remember that, I love all of you.

I welcome your correspondence at:
author.kvincent@gmail.com

Thank you

www.ingramcontent.com/pod-product-compliance
Lightning Source LLC
Chambersburg PA
CBHW072255310526
45795CB00012B/1415